On Being a Veterinarian

Book 3:

Practicing Small Animal Medicine

April Kung, DVM

Content disclaimer: Any incidents recounted in this series that are based on true occurrences have had select details altered to protect confidentiality. Suggestions made are based on the author's personal experience and research. Author claims no professional training or education in financial or legal matters, psychiatry, psychology, human nutrition, exercise physiology, or medical education. Please consult a certified or licensed expert in these areas for professional help. Any advice on veterinary medical practice provided by the author is intended for application by licensed veterinarians capable of using their own medical judgment. Do not attempt to use any medical advice provided by the author without a medical degree. In no event should the author be responsible or liable, directly or indirectly, for any damage or loss caused or alleged to be caused by, or in connection with, the use of or reliance on any such information provided by the author. Health-related topics, legal and financial information provided by the author should not be substituted for professional medical, legal and financial advice. It is your responsibility to research the accuracy, completeness and usefulness of all opinions and other information provided by the author. The author assumes no responsibility or liability for any consequence resulting, directly or indirectly, for any action or inaction taken based on or made in reliance on the information provided.

Published by Happy Animal Productions
First Edition January 2018
ISBN-13: 978-1-948356-04-6

This book is dedicated to my father.
Dad, I wish you could have made it to Flagstaff.

Table of Contents

Preface

Before reading this or any of the other books in this series, please download and read the free *Book Series Introduction* from my website. It explains the aim and scope of the *On Being a Veterinarian Series*, including who the series is for, and perhaps more importantly, who it's not for. Additional help and advice for future veterinarians is available on my website at www.realize.vet

One of my favorite medical satire websites is GomerBlog. A couple years ago it featured an article entitled, *"Optimistic, Bright-Eyed Med Students Eager to Transform into Jaded, Burned-Out Physicians."* The article describes the moment when medical students, "bursting with altruism" and "full of dreams" "break out of their optimistic cocoons [...] and morph into creatures of unbridled pessimism and apathy." In the article, a psychiatrist asserts that this jadedness is "a sign of a truly mature physician." An internal medicine residency program director adds that when this transformation takes place, "That's when I know I can call you my colleague."[10]

Humorous as this article is, there is truth in it. I began my veterinary career bright-eyed and optimistic. During my first six months of mentorship at the ER where I was hired after vet school, everything was exciting and fun. However, I detected mild irritation in some of my more experienced colleagues. My enthusiasm seemed to irk them. This was a barrier between us and it prevented any sense of camaraderie. A year later however, after my optimism had been stripped away by the realities of practice, by transition shock, I felt more accepted by the other doctors. They began to treat me as a colleague.

Later in my career, the tables were turned. I was the experienced veterinarian when a new graduate was hired by my hospital. The light of a thousand suns shined from her happy eyes. Her enthusiasm irked me. As the months passed though, the light in her eyes gradually dimmed. Gone was the naïve optimism. Reality had set in. Now we were truly colleagues. I wish I could have done better for her. I wish I could have been a better mentor. But she was just so enthusiastic... And I was just so jaded.

It isn't that experienced doctors wish ill on the idealistic newcomers to this field. We don't derive secret satisfaction from seeing that enthusiasm die. It's simply that the exuberant new graduate is still living in a land of mirages, where perfect medicine is practiced, where we solve every medical mystery and nothing bad ever happens. She hasn't yet been disillusioned of her illusions, and until she has, we don't exist in the same dimension, we don't speak the same language and we have little in common. Perhaps also, we jaded practitioners are irritated by the bright-eyed optimism of the new graduate because we are still grieving the loss of our own naive optimism.

I'd like to eradicate the dichotomy between the enthusiastic new graduate and the jaded, seasoned practitioner. The transition from the former to the latter currently involves falling from a great height as the unrealistic expectations of the new graduate are pulled from beneath his feet. The injuries sustained from this fall can cause permanent damage, and that sense of enthusiasm for veterinary medicine can be lost forever.

The early sections of the book were written with the hope of helping you enter the field with greater sobriety. You may not fall at all, and so you may never descend into jaded apathy. Perhaps instead, you'll find the happy medium between realism and enthusiasm that we all seek. What I really hope is that when you become the seasoned practitioner, you'll meet nothing but sober yet realistically enthusiastic new graduates, and you'll immediately feel you can call them colleagues.

Later in the book, I provide practical tips for helping you become an astute and effective practitioner, without paying the emotional toll of learning everything the hard way. These discussions unveil some of the common underlying day to day challenges of clinical practice.

Unlike human medicine, where the standards and protocols are more clear cut, veterinary medicine is still a bit like the old wild west. If you ask ten different veterinarians for an opinion on how to practice medicine, you may get ten different answers. Bear this in mind as you read, and ask other veterinarians for their opinions on the topics covered in this book. The more perspectives you get, the greater the breadth of options you'll have to choose from when it comes time for you to decide how you want to practice veterinary medicine - and it is for you to decide. Never forget that.

The last sections of the book offer information to help you decide where to begin your career, and additional options to consider as you gain more experience. Perhaps most importantly, I give you the foresight to know how to choose a good employer. I provide a list of the top skills employers want in new graduate veterinarians so you can proactively work on these skills as a veterinary student, and I suggest other things you can do to make yourself a good investment for your employer. Also included is some logistical information I wish I'd had as a new graduate.

Before You
Become a Doctor

Sit somewhere quiet where you won't be disturbed or distracted. Close your eyes, and spend at least ten minutes imagining in vivid detail exactly what you want your life as a small animal veterinarian to look like. Where do you live? What does your house look like? Do you have a yard? A garden? What kind of people do you work with? What kind of hospital do you work at? What's your boss like? What are your fellow doctors like? What kind of relationship do you have with them? What's your personality as a doctor? How do you feel every day while you're at work?

What does your personal life look like? What kind of things do you do to take care of your body and mind? What kinds of hobbies do you have? Where do you go for vacations? What do you do on those vacations? Is there someone wonderful sharing your life? What is he or she like? What kinds of friends do you have? Do you have kids? Pets? How much time do you get to spend with the important people and animals in your life? What kinds of emotions are you experiencing day to day in this future ideal life of yours? Joy? Fulfillment? Optimism?

After you've got a crystal clear vision in your mind about your future as a veterinary doctor, cement it in your brain by re-envisioning it on a regular basis. Do it while you're having your morning coffee or tea. The reason I want you to hold onto this vision is so that you can use it as a compass. If, after you become a veterinarian, you find yourself living a life that doesn't resemble what you envisioned for yourself, remember your original vision and use it to navigate out of the life you don't want and into the life you do. While our futures rarely (if ever) turn out to be exactly what we envision - and the practice of medicine especially likes to confound our perfect plans - if we are clear in advance about what we want the flavor and the spirit of our future lives to be, we are far more likely to find ourselves living an approximation of that vision. But, if we don't have a clear vision in advance, it's all too easy to end up tolerating the kind of life we shouldn't. In my opinion, too many veterinarians are tolerating what they shouldn't. That is not the future I want for you.

When You Become a Doctor

There are two things I want you to do either before or immediately after you begin practicing. First, seek out other newly graduated veterinarians in your area. Run an ad on Craigslist, in the local paper, in your state or city veterinary medical association newsletter. Start a group. Meet on a regular basis. Meet for drinks, or coffee, or pie, or meet virtually via a group call on Skype. Share with each other your experiences and perceptions as new vets. Compare notes about the different hospitals where you all work. Talk about difficult cases you've seen or issues you're facing. This can accelerate learning for all of you, as well as providing the critical, empathetic social support all of you will need, and that you can't really get from people who don't walk in your shoes. Take care to prevent these meetings from becoming opportunities merely to complain. You should all feel that you can talk about negative things that have happened, but the goal should be combating feelings of isolation and helping each other deal with the negatives in a constructive way.

The second thing I want you to do is to find a psychiatrist. Yes, even if you feel perfectly fine. As a new veterinarian, the time to start seeing a good psychiatrist is before you need one. You may need to see several before you find one you click with. Tell them you're a recent graduate of veterinary school, you've heard the first several years of practice can be tough and you want to be proactive about your own mental health. See how they respond. When you find one who "gets it," see them on a regular basis - at least monthly, and at least for the first year, but preferably for your first five years in practice.

Why a psychiatrist? Because when you begin practicing, in addition to your support group of other new grads, I want you to have a therapist who knows what it's like to practice medicine. Psychiatrists are MDs. Their friends are MDs. They know firsthand how difficult medical practice can be, especially when you're just starting out. The other reason I recommend seeing a psychiatrist is because they can prescribe medications for depression and anxiety. You may never need these medications, but if you do, it's nice not to have to schedule more appointments with someone else. You're going to be busy. Every hour of free time is precious.

The Honest Imposter?

You are a doctor. You have the education, the degree and your state license. It's day one of your first job. You're all decked out in a brand new white coat and there's a stethoscope around your neck. Your coat pockets contain bandage scissors, a pair of hemostats, tweezers, a magnifying glass, and the notebook you call your medical bible in which you've listed emergency drug doses, IV fluid calculation formulae, the cranial nerves and their functions, and pretty much every other piece of information you think you might need to access quickly.

You're excited but you're also scared. You know it's important to appear confident to clients and coworkers so you're masking all your doubts and worries under a façade of relaxed congeniality. But what if you do something wrong? What if you can't remember something really important? At this moment, getting ready to see your first client, you're pretty sure you don't remember anything. What if you can't correctly interpret a radiograph or a chemistry panel? What will the other doctors think of you? Will the technicians lose respect for you? Are you truly good enough and smart enough to be a doctor? What if a client asks you how long you've been practicing? You can't lie. You'll have to tell them you've just started. What if they don't want you to be their pet's doctor because you're too inexperienced? What if none of the clients want you to be their veterinarian because it will be obvious you have no idea what you're doing?

These are normal thoughts stemming from Imposter Syndrome, which I describe in Book 2. It's okay. Every new doctor feels this way. In fact most of us feel this way for the first several years. Yup. *Years*. I had a dialogue similar to this running non-stop through my mind the entire time I worked as an emergency vet. I worried constantly that clients would grill me about my experience, that the other doctors at my hospital thought I was stupid, that my diagnostic and treatment plans revealed the depths of my ineptitude and that everyone was meeting in private to talk about how it was a mistake to have hired me. I was sure at some point I would get called into the medical director's office and he would tell me I was an awful doctor and then fire me.

It's only in the last couple years that I've felt confident enough in my abilities as a veterinarian to start being honest about my feelings of self-doubt. Want to know what I've discovered? Every other doctor I've ever talked to feels the same way and went through the same miserable terror when they first started practicing. Every. Single. One. When my husband first started working as a "real doctor," he too experienced this fear and self doubt.

I hope telling you how universal these thoughts are will help when you step into your real doctor shoes. I remember feeling incredibly alone – inside my head it was just me and all these terrified, paranoid, negative, self-flagellating thoughts, while on the outside I pretended to be confident and ready to take on the world. Every time I scrubbed in for an emergency surgery in the middle of the night, I would chat casually with the technicians while under the surface a writhing snake pit of self-recrimination hissed at me, "you should not be doing this." Secretly, I begged the spirit of my mother, who passed away when I was in vet school, to help me perform the surgery correctly and without harming my patient.

I was inexperienced, so of course I made mistakes. A lot of them. Some of them small and inconsequential, but some of them big and devastating. Some of them, perhaps, could have been prevented had I been honest about my fears and asked for more help. Every error added more fuel to the self-doubt and fear that consumed me. Looking back on those first few years, I honestly don't know how I was able to keep going. How did I will myself out of bed and continue going to work despite the suffocating terror inside? I remember sitting in the doctors' office before my shift, fearing I would find out in doctors' rounds of yet another mistake I'd made, fearing that the night would bring terrors I could not handle. To calm myself, I'd listen to Shawn Mullin's song *Lullaby* as he sang "everything is gonna' be alright"- over and over again.

I don't want you to feel this way when you begin your career. It was Imposter Syndrome and the fear of being found wanting that kept me hiding inside my head and living that lonely misery for years. Don't do that. It's okay to say you've never done something before and you don't feel comfortable doing it alone. It's okay to be honest about your fears and self-doubts. It's okay to ask another doctor for help interpreting a radiograph or chemistry panel. It's okay to let your technicians see that you're a human being just starting out in a very difficult career and to ask for their help. One of my classmates had a great way of asking the technicians she worked with for help. She would ask, "What would the other doctors do in this situation?"

And if, when you start your first job, a client asks how long you've been practicing, just tell them the truth – from one human being to another - and let the cards fall where they may. Say it with a smile, and say it like it's the wonderful, amazing thing that it is. Say it as if speaking to a good friend, with the expectation that they will be as excited as you are. "Today is my first day!"

If another doctor or a member of the support staff gives you a hard time about not knowing something, just say, "Yes, before I started vet school I thought I would know everything when I graduated. Now I realize that's impossible. I know I still have a lot to learn, but I'm doing the best I can, and with your help, hopefully I'll get better every day." Then look into their eyes, and smile.

You are not an imposter. You are a doctor. Even when you're afraid. Even when you're imperfect. Even when you make mistakes. Even when the technicians know things you don't. Even when clients question you. Even when you you're not sure what to do. You are still a doctor, and every day you practice you will become a better doctor - and every experienced doctor knows this - so there is nothing to be ashamed of and there is nothing to hide.

Even if you practiced for a hundred years, you couldn't know all there is to know. You'd still feel uncertain about some of your diagnoses and treatments. The only difference would be that you'd have gained the confidence and the courage to be honest about your self-doubts. It takes enormous courage to wear that white coat - to take on the responsibilities of a veterinary doctor. Why not push yourself to exude one tiny drop more of that courage? Go ahead and just be honest from day one. You can't be an imposter if you're honest. I'm not saying you should wear all your fears on your sleeve and walk around like an energy sucking Eeyore. I'm saying stand up straight and wear that white coat with pride - because you earned it - but also wear it with the honest humility that all good doctors have. We are all still learning.

The Slow Turtle

During my early days of working as an ER vet, when I was still within my six month mentorship window, a dog was brought in for abnormal behavior. My medical director went to talk to the dog's owners, but sent the dog back to the treatment area for me to examine. The dog overreacted when I tested his pupillary reflexes, and his pupils were enlarged and slow to respond to my flashlight. More worryingly, he was having difficulty walking and was dribbling urine as he faltered about.

I racked my brain for what could be causing these signs. I rifled through the quick reference notebook - what I call my "medical bible" - that I started creating when I was a fourth year vet student. (A video to help you create your own medical bible is available at www.realize.vet/book3-resources.) Here's a picture of the page I consulted.

BLADDER INNERVATION

[L1-2] Hypogastric N. (Sympathetic)   [S1-3] Pudendal N. (Somatic)

Pelvic N. (parasymp & sensory)

β = relax detrusor
Muscarinic = Contract
— bethanecol detrusor
— metoclopramide
α = constrict
Ach = constrict

Internal Sphincter   External Sphincter

Hypocontractile bladder (α-antagonist)
— LMN dz
— Detrusor atony
Rx para-mimetics (metoclopramide, bethanecol), Cisapride

Hypercontractile bladder
— UMN dz — detrusor instability
Rx anticholinergics or β-mimetics
• Propantheline, oxybutynin • terbutaline
Oxytriol Dicyclomine

α-agonists
— phenylpropanolamine (PPA)
DES (diethylstilbesterol)
α-blockers
— Prazosin
— Phenoxybenzamine
— Tamsulosin (select α)

Hypertonic urethra
— UMN dz, urethral spasm, dysergia
Rx α-antag: Prazosin, phenoxybenzamine
Sk m relax: Diazepam, Dantrolene

Hypotonic urethra
— Smt, spay incont.
Rx α-agonists
pseudoephedrine, PPA or Hormones
DES or GnRH & methyltestosterone &

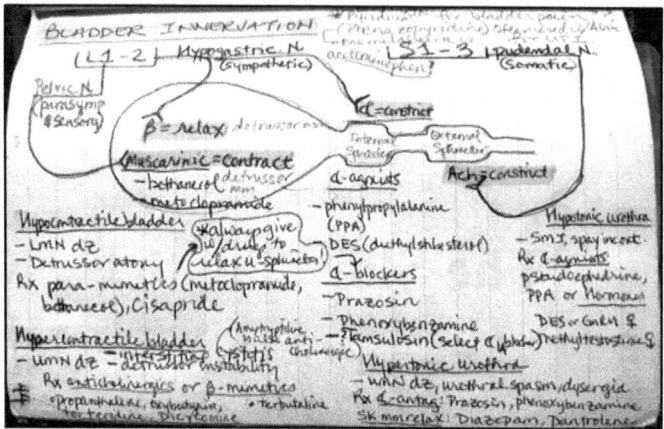

Okay, let's see. The nerves to the urinary bladder and the external and internal urinary sphincters are the pelvic nerve, the hypogastric nerve and the pudendal nerve. Both the hypogastric and pudendal nerves cause constriction of the sphincters – so there could be something wrong with those nerves, and that would explain why urine was dribbling out. Those two nerves emerge from the sacral and the lumbar spine. Could there be an abnormality in the lower spine affecting both these nerves?

But what about the dog's difficulty walking? It's not confined to just his hind legs. All four of his legs are affected. If the problem is related to the spinal cord, it would have to be way up in his neck, in his cervical spine, in order to explain deficiencies in all four limbs. But neither of those explanations are consistent with his slow pupillary reflexes. Therefore, the problem must be in his brain. What part of the brain would have to be affected in order to cause all these different symptoms?

I was very worried about this dog. There must be something terribly wrong. A brain tumor perhaps. But where? The abnormal pupillary reflexes indicated a problem in the forebrain or the midbrain, but bladder control could be affected by the forebrain or the hindbrain. Neurological abnormalities causing deficiencies in all four limbs could also be attributed to the brain. What was it the Neurology Professor said in vet school? The more abnormal the gait, the further back in the brain the lesion is likely to be?

As I was standing there, my eyes growing wider as my conviction increased that something horrible must be affecting multiple areas of this dog's brain, my medical director came back to the treatment area. As we both watched this poor animal stumble around, dripping urine all over the floor, I told him of my physical exam findings and gave him a brief recap of my diagnostic reasoning. He chuckled. I was shocked. Didn't he care that something awful was wrong with this dog? Why was he so relaxed?

He turned to me and asked, "What would you say if I told you this dog was brought in by two teenage boys who are both acting strange?"

I shook my head back at him. I had no idea.

"This dog is high," he said, chuckling some more. "He got into their marijuana."

Aha! Marijuana effects multiple areas of the brain including the forebrain (which could explain the slowed pupillary reflexes and loss of urinary control) and the part of the brain involved in balance and coordination (which explained the dog's difficulty walking).

"Did they tell you that?" I asked, sure that was the only way he could have solved this case so quickly.

"No, but I've seen this a dozen times."

This, in a nutshell, is the difference between a new veterinarian and an experienced veterinarian. Since I had never seen a case of marijuana toxicity before, I was using an analytic approach that drew on what I'd learned of "elaborate causal networks" of "pathophysiological processes." This is a perfectly respectable method for diagnostic reasoning. It just makes you feel as slow as a turtle, and it has the potential to send you down a few blind alleys - which makes you feel like an even slower turtle.

My medical director, who had "seen this a dozen times," had used pattern recognition, which is much faster. He wasn't thinking about the pathophysiological explanations at all. He didn't have to. Thanks to his previous experiences with similar cases, he instantly recognized the pattern of clinical signs that manifest in dogs exposed to marijuana. This is one justification for making interns and medical residents work such long hours and see so many cases. "Extensive exposure to many different cases may be the critical factor in developing expertise."[18] Pattern recognition is the cornerstone of clinical expertise.

But if you look back at the analytical reasoning I did on the case of the stumbling, urinating dog, you'll realize that I actually did come to the correct conclusion. The dog's problem was indeed in multiple areas of his brain. And after my medical director revealed that marijuana toxicity was the cause, I never again forgot that toxicity should be at the top of my list of suspicions whenever symptoms of diffuse brain abnormalities are present. And I've certainly never forgotten what a dog who's high on marijuana acts like. That case greatly enhanced my arsenal of pattern recognition, and I solved subsequent similar cases much more quickly.

This isn't to say say, however, that once you become an experienced clinician you'll never use the analytical approach again. Pattern recognition is a necessary ingredient of clinical expertise, but in and of itself, it's not sufficient. If pattern recognition alone were enough, a veterinary assistant or technician with years of experience could be a doctor. Pattern recognition can help rule out unlikely diagnoses quickly and shorten the list of possible diagnoses, but it must still be combined with a doctor's knowledge of patholophysiological processes to make a definitive diagnosis. When a medical case is straightforward, you can make a diagnosis based on pattern recognition so long as everything about the case is consistent with your knowledge of pathophysiological processes. But when a medical case isn't straightforward, pattern recognition also has the potential to send you down blind alleys.

Consider this example. A patient presents with difficulty breathing. Pulse oximetry confirms abnormally low levels of oxygen in the blood. A heart murmur and crackling sounds are heard when a stethoscope is used to listen to the patient's chest. Chest radiographs show a pattern consistent with fluid overload in the lungs. This could be a slam dunk case of heart failure.

Pattern recognition combines the following observations to make the diagnosis of heart failure:

1. Respiratory distress
2. Low blood oxygen content
3. A heart murmur
4. Crackling sounds from fluid in the lungs
5. Chest radiographs consistent with fluid overload in the lungs

After seeing this combination a few times, almost anyone would be able to diagnose heart failure - and in many cases, they'd be right. In *many* cases - but not all. If the patient responds to treatment for acute heart failure and breathing improves, pattern recognition has enabled a quick diagnosis and effective symptom resolution. But what if the patient is treated for acute heart failure yet breathing and blood oxygenation don't improve? This is where continued dependence on pattern recognition ceases to be helpful and could even potentially be harmful. Only the slower, analytical approach using the doctor's knowledge of pathophysiological processes has a chance of leading to the correct diagnosis.

Here's a simplified summary of the pathophysiological processes underlying acute heart failure: A heart murmur can indicate underlying heart disease. If heart disease is present and the heart is too weak to do its job of pumping blood, blood backs up behind the heart, just like cars back up when a traffic light is broken. If blood can't move forward through the arterial system like it's supposed to, pressure increases in the veins behind the heart. Eventually enough pressure builds up to push blood plasma (the liquid portion of the blood that does not contain red blood cells) through the semi-porous membranes of the tiny blood vessels in the lungs - resulting in the fluid overload in the lungs that causes respiratory distress.

Acute heart failure is typically treated with an intravenous injection of furosemide, which is a diuretic. This drug causes increased blood flow to the kidneys and increased fluid excretion through the kidneys. Urination reduces the amount of fluid in the blood vessels, thereby reducing fluid overload in the lungs. If the diuretic fails to induce urination however, the doctor must consider whether there is something wrong with the kidneys.

Perhaps the heart murmur is just a red herring. The kidneys filter blood and excrete excess fluid. If they aren't functioning and the patient isn't producing any urine, that too can cause fluid overload in the body - and in the lungs. If blood chemistry reveals abnormally elevated kidney values, the more likely cause of the patient's fluid overload then becomes acute kidney failure. The doctor must then then use her knowledge of pathophysiological processes to determine what available medical treatments might be effective in reducing fluid overload if the patient can't be made to urinate.

So you see, pattern recognition can make a doctor faster, but it's the analytical approach and knowledge of pathophysiological processes that make a doctor a doctor. When you begin practicing, you're going to feel like a turtle compared to your more experienced colleagues. You may even notice that support staff seem to come to conclusions more quickly than you do. New veterinarians often observe their comparative lack of speed and conclude there's something wrong with them. They feel inadequate and proceed to doubt their worth as doctors. But now you'll know that your lack of speed is no reflection of a lack of knowledge nor a lack or worth. It's merely a lack of simple pattern recognition, and that's nothing to beat yourself up about because pattern recognition comes to all of us the same way - one case at a time.

The article referenced in this passage has some great information about how medical expertise develops. As of this writing, it's available free on the internet. Just Google *A Cognitive Perspective on Medical Expertise* by H.G. Schmidt, Ph.D., or go to www.realize.vet/book3-resources for a direct link.

The Beautiful Mirage

"Enjoy the journey, because the destination is a mirage."
- Steven Furtik

When Alex and I moved to Flagstaff for his job, I gave my elderly father the option to move here too. He was wheelchair bound and in poor physical condition, but he was very enthusiastic about moving. He looked forward to all the adventures awaiting him in this new place with its wonderful scenery and year round sunshine. Before we moved my father though, we wanted to build a handicap accessible apartment for him. My father's place in Illinois was not handicap friendly, and since both front and back entrances had stairs, my father only left his apartment for doctor appointments.

The place we were creating for him in Flagstaff would have no stairs. It would have a little patio outside a set of extra wide French doors so he would be able to just roll out anytime he liked. My father was elated about this. He planned to have a little garden on his patio to grow his favorite vegetables and herbs.

His local library had a delivery service and he ordered dozens of books on gardening. When I called to check on him he was always excited to tell me new things he was learning regarding the best soil fertilizers or innovative techniques for protecting garden vegetables from insect pests. I pictured my father outside on his patio, leaning forward in his wheelchair to water his precious plants. I saw him sitting in the bright sunlight with his white hair looking almost translucent as he listened to birdsong and gazed at the snow covered peaks of Mount Elden.

He would arrive just in time to see a magical, white Christmas in Flagstaff. I decorated the pine tree in front of his patio with Christmas ornaments and twinkling lights. But he suffered a massive stroke and died one month before his scheduled move. I told my sister I felt crushed by the guilt of leaving him alone in Illinois for almost a year while creating this place that he would never get to enjoy. "But he did get to enjoy it," she said. "He spent the last year of his life happily fantasizing about a beautiful and perfect future, and the future we imagine is almost always better than the real thing turns out to be."

My sister's words were a great comfort to me, and they helped me see from a perspective I hadn't before. Before he died, my father talked incessantly about growing tropical papaya trees on his patio in Flagstaff.

Despite my repeated admonishments that papaya trees can't grow in Flagstaff because it's 7,000 feet above sea level and the climate won't support them, every time I telephoned my father, he talked about his future papaya trees. I told him he could grow certain kinds of apple trees here, but not papayas. He wouldn't listen. It made me so frustrated. But now I'm glad he didn't listen to me. I'm glad he kept on dreaming about his mirage of papaya trees. It made him happy. It's just a little paradoxical if you think about it though. Had he lived he would have been disappointed.

I can't think of a single example in my life where things turned out as I thought they would. Wherever it is we think we're headed is really just a made up picture that exists only in our heads - a beautiful mirage. Since we can't see the future, we project these pretty pictures over the open highway that lies before us - and even though "the future we imagine is almost always better than the real thing turns out to be" – our projections bring us joy in the present and inspire us to keep moving forward.

I'm torn by this paradox. On the one hand, I want to protect you from later disillusionment. Whether you dream of being a DVM or an MD or a DO or a DPM or a DDS, the entire field of medicine is littered with mirages. On the other hand, I don't want to deprive you of the pleasure and the passion of envisioning a beautiful future for yourself as a doctor.

So here's what I'm going to do: I'm going to reveal the two most important mirages in veterinary medicine, but I'm not going to leave you without a vision to aim for. I'm going to exchange the mirages for the more realistic future you can look forward to. The caveat is that we're trading illusion for reality, so what I'm offering isn't as bewitching as the mirages. I'm replacing the papayas (mirage) with apples (reality).

Why should you let me take these pretty medical mirages from you? Because they're dangerous to future doctors. The moment you step into one, it will turn to quicksand. I'd much rather you start your career knowing the facts of where you're headed, and standing squarely on solid ground.

Papaya #1: Gold Standard Veterinary Medicine

If you do most of your fourth year rotations at a teaching hospital, you'll get to see the most advanced tests and treatments available. There will be echocardiograms with Doppler color flow and endoscopies with intestinal biopsies. There will be spinal taps and blood gas analyses. You'll get to watch as CT scans and MRIs are performed and interpreted. You'll get to assist during spinal surgeries, hip replacements, pacemaker implantations, cholecystectomies, and thoracic duct ligations. You'll see chemotherapy and radiation therapy and maybe even brain surgery. The thrill of partaking in the process of coming to a correct diagnosis, and of seeing patients improve with the right treatments, will fill you with a euphoric, swelling sensation in your chest that feels just like falling in love, and you'll think that's what it's going to be like when you start practicing. But this is a mirage.

Unless you pursue specialization and teach in an academic hospital, or start your career in a first-rate private specialty hospital, you will never again approach the perfect medicine that enthralled you in the teaching hospital. It will glimmer and beckon to you from the ever receding horizon behind you. Resource availability between different veterinary hospitals outside of academia varies immensely. The facilities and human resources at the private emergency hospital where I started my veterinary career were meager compared to the seemingly unlimited resources of my teaching hospital, but they were far superior to those of the many day practices and other emergency hospitals where I would later work. Many of those hospitals didn't even carry broad spectrum intravenous antibiotics, some didn't have good pain medications like morphine, a couple of them had no ultrasound machine, and one had no dental drill, no ophthalmoscope or surgical gowns, and their head technician was unable to perform venipuncture.

Limitations vary by hospital, geographical location, demographics, and the state of the economy, obviously, but my point is that what you get taught in vet school and see in the teaching hospital is not the kind of medicine that gets practiced outside of academia or the very best specialty centers. Unfortunately, what you most need to know about practicing veterinary medicine in the real world isn't taught at all. Veterinary schools absolutely should and must teach gold standard medicine, but cram packed with information as the curriculum already is, there simply isn't time for them to also teach the myriad possible compromised diagnostic and treatment plan combinations used in the enormous expanse of the veterinary medicine universe outside of academia.

Limited resources in private hospitals won't be the only barrier to practicing Gold Standard Veterinary Medicine. As a fourth year vet student doing your clinical rotations in a teaching hospital, virtually every pet owner you meet will be both able and willing to pursue advanced diagnostics and treatments for their pets. Outside the veterinary teaching hospital, when a case is complicated and you lack resources or expertise, you'll want to recommend a specialty consult for the sake of the pet. Unless you work in an affluent area though, you'll find that on average only about half your clients can or will follow this recommendation. This means you will have to muddle through as best you can, usually on a shoestring budget. Even for the more straightforward cases that you do feel confident managing, few clients simply say "okay, doctor" after you present a cost estimate with your gold standard medical recommendations.

So what do you do when the gold standard you learned can't be applied? When you've finally put the millions of separate puzzle pieces of your medical knowledge together in the right configuration, which pieces do you remove when a pet owner says "No"? In the movie *Amadeus,* the king tells Mozart that his piano concerto has "too many notes," and he should cut a few out. Mozart retorts, "Which few did you have in mind, Majesty?" Just like the notes in Mozart's masterpiece, every component of a gold standard medical recommendation has a reason for being, and just like the king in *Amadeus*, few pet owners understand this. I once had a pet owner say to me, "Why do we have to do all these tests? Can't you just tell me what's wrong?"

Diagnosing a medical problem is serious detective work. The patient's symptoms are clues, but since our patients can't talk, we have to take what clients report with a grain of salt. If a client says his dog is coughing, is the dog truly coughing or is he gagging? If a pet owner brings her indoor-outdoor cat to the hospital because he isn't eating, is that true or can we be sure he doesn't just prefer the food the neighbors are leaving out for him? If a client says her pet was prescribed a round, white pill by a different veterinarian, was it an antibiotic or a pain medication? A good, thorough physical exam can yield better clues, but even so, you don't solve a mystery case based only on clues.

You need evidence, and not just one piece of evidence. A single piece of evidence can be used to support many different theories, so by itself it's rarely sufficient to prove anything. Sometimes a single piece of evidence is wrong. Remember the false negatives and false positives I told you about in Book 2? It might be an anomaly or a machine error. Maybe we think it's evidence but it doesn't have anything at all to do with the case. This is why, just like a crime scene investigation, we need multiple pieces of evidence all pointing toward the same conclusion before we can be confident we've identified the right culprit. Evidence comes from diagnostic tests, and every diagnostic test gives us different pieces of evidence.

A complete blood count (CBC) tells us whether the pet is anemic, and what kind of anemia it is. Maybe it's from an iron deficiency. Maybe it's because of an acute hemorrhage. We also get to find out how anemic a patient is. Mild, moderate or severe? This information has a huge impact on how we proceed. A CBC tells us whether the platelets, which are a necessary part of the blood clotting process, are normal or low. If they're abnormally low, are they the primary problem or is this secondary to a bleed somewhere? A white blood cell count is a part of the CBC as well. White blood cells are immune cells and when a patient is sick, It's important to know whether the immune cells are high, low or normal.

A chemistry panel tells us about the health of some different organs in the body, like the kidneys and the liver. Both of these organs play a part in drug metabolism and excretion. Having an idea of how these organs are functioning can help us know how much or little of a drug should be prescribed, or whether certain drugs should be prescribed at all. A chemistry panel also lets us evaluate blood proteins like albumin. If albumin is low, it can mean there has been a bleed, or that kidney or GI disease may be present. Knowing the albumin level is also important in deciding what fluid therapy regimen we should use. We get vital information about a patient's electrolyte values from a chemistry panel too. Electrolyte abnormalities by themselves can be life threatening if severe. If we attempt to treat a sick patient without knowing these values we could end up causing even more harm. Certain electrolyte abnormalities are very helpful in pointing us toward a definitive diagnosis. The chemistry panel also tells us whether the patient's blood glucose is normal, low or high. This can tell us if we're dealing with dangerous conditions like diabetic ketoacidosis or hypoglycemia, both of which can be fatal if not treated promptly and correctly.

A urinalysis or UA first of all tells us the animal is producing some urine, which is very important to know. The UA can help us diagnose a urinary tract infection, or it may indicate there is a cancerous tumor inside the bladder. It could tell us if the abnormal kidney values on the chemistry panel are more likely due to dehydration or kidney disease. A UA can also be used to confirm a diagnosis of diabetic ketoacidosis.

Chest x-rays can help us determine whether a coughing patient has heart disease, pneumonia, lung cancer, bronchitis, or even an esophageal foreign body obstruction – each of these requires a different treatment. They can help us figure out if there is fluid building up in the sac around the heart, or if there is fluid or air building up outside the lungs. Both of these conditions can be fatal and require different types of emergency intervention.

Abdominal x-rays can show whether any of the abdominal organs are enlarged, displaced, abnormally shaped, or filled with air. They can help diagnose an infection in the uterus, a gastrointestinal blockage or bladder stones, all of which require surgery. Abdominal ultra sound can help us differentiate between pregnancy and an infection in the uterus, or confirm there is fluid in the abdomen and a suspicious mass on the spleen. We can use ultrasound to examine the inner architecture of organs like the kidneys, the urinary bladder, the spleen, the liver, and the gall bladder.

These are just some of the most common diagnostic tests, and only some of the important information they can yield. There are catalogs full of different kinds of diagnostic tests. Many need to be performed in addition to the tests already mentioned to get a definitive diagnosis. Often we need to repeat our initial diagnostic tests in order to know whether our treatments are helping or not.

The list of things that could be wrong with a sick patient is intimidatingly long. So when a client only has enough money to do one test, which one do you do? Perhaps the client has so little money there will only be enough for the exam fee plus some basic treatment. But if you don't know what's wrong with the patient, what treatment do you prescribe? This is what they don't teach you in vet school: How to make do when Gold Standard Veterinary Medicine is not an option.

Apple #1: The Joy of Making Do

Last week after a pretty rigorous 10 mile hike in the outback of Arizona, Alex and I were relieved to get back to his truck just as the sun had set. He'd bought a used, lifted Chevy Suburban specifically so we could take the rugged off-roads way back into the wilderness to explore the most remote trails. It was a new moon so there was little light. We were glad to have the bright off-road lights of the truck to illuminate the seven miles of rocky 4x4-only road we had to traverse before reaching the main road. Temperatures in the desert can drop quickly after sunset and my sweat soaked clothes exacerbated the chill seeping into my bones. I was very happy to have the truck's cabin heat on full blast.

After climbing one of the first big boulders on the road, the truck came down the other side with an ominous "clunk." At first we thought the boulder had hit the undercarriage of the truck, which wouldn't necessarily result in serious damage, but just to be sure, Alex stopped the truck and we both got out to look. In the bright lights shining from the roof of the truck we could see that the top of the right front tire was tilted inward at a 45 degree angle. My heart sank. I don't know a lot about cars but when one of your wheels falls off it seems a given you're going to need some professional help. I was certain we would have to hike the seven rocky miles to the main road despite the cold and darkness, and despite our exhaustion. There would be no cellular service until we reached the main road. And after that long, unpleasant walk, we would still have to wait hours for a specialized 4x4 tow truck before we could even think of getting somewhere warm to shed our clammy clothes.

Alex figured out that the ball joint of the right suspension arm had failed. A ball joint is similar to a hip joint. If you Google images of hip joints online, you'll see how the round head of the femur is supposed to fit snuggly within the concave acetabulum. So in essence, one of the truck's hip joints had become dislocated – the ball had popped out of its housing completely. These joints are designed to fit so snuggly they have to be reduced by a machine press in a factory. When they fail - you don't try to fix them. You replace them. Still, Alex felt it was worth at least trying to reduce the dislocated ball joint. Worst case scenario: He'd fail and we'd have to walk to the main road. If he didn't try at all, we'd have to walk to the main road anyway, so - what the heck.

He reasoned that if he jacked up the front of the truck and aligned the two pieces of the joint perfectly, when he lowered the truck, its weight would be enough to force the ball back into its housing. I helped by turning the steering wheel left and right as he instructed from outside the truck. Over the course of an hour and a half, he must have raised and lowered this 3-ton truck twenty times, but that joint would just not pop back together. He was about to give up when he came up with what he called a "Hail Mary" idea.

He had a ratchet strap in the back of the truck. Maybe,

if the ratchet strap was strong enough, he could wrap it around the two disconnected parts of the joint and slowly ratchet them together until the ball popped into place. With another loud "clunk" he successfully reduced the joint. For several moments, the two of just sat there in stunned disbelief. It seemed too good to be true. Alex had fixed what was theoretically unfixable using nothing more than a jack and a ratchet strap. We had to drive very slowly to ensure the ball didn't pop back out of its housing but we were able to limp the truck to the main road and all the way back home because of Alex's brilliant improvisation. "There can be no true joy without adversity," he said as we headed home. When I asked him what he meant, he explained that fixing the truck by creatively making do gave him a feeling of pride and satisfaction that he never could have gained if he'd had a brand new ball joint on hand.

When I remember my happiest moments of genuine pride, it's always been because I figured out a novel solution to a problem using just what was available to me in the moment. Last week one of the arms of my reading glasses fell off and I couldn't find the pin. I tried using a paper clip instead of the pin to re-secure the arm in place but the pin hole was too small. I looked around my office to see what random tool might help me solve this problem. When my eyes fell upon a Bic lighter, I knew I had the solution. I used the lighter to heat and soften the plastic around the pin hole while I pushed the paperclip through, and voila – my glasses were fixed.

This is what makes being a human being so much fun.

I don't think many things in life can bring us a better sense of accomplishment and self-respect than regularly using our noggins to make do with what we've got. When we get the chance to innovate, we get to express our creativity. We get reminded of our own ingenuity, and it feels great.

When I compare my perceptions as a new veterinarian to those I hold now on the topic of practicing veterinary medicine, they're like night and day. As a new vet, I felt it was my personal duty to push myself, my support staff and my clients to adhere to the gold standards. Even though the resources to do this were clearly lacking, practicing below the gold standard felt dirty to me. There was a persistent squeezing sensation around my chest. I felt like I was doing something wrong, and all my vet school professors could see me and were disgusted with how I was degrading myself and the profession.

I worried myself sick over every single medical case in which I couldn't perform every diagnostic test or prescribe every treatment I thought I should. I was convinced any deviation from the gold standard would trigger a physiological pathway to doom like some kind of grisly Rube Goldberg machine. The end of that unfortunate chain of events would be my patient's death, the loss of my job and maybe even my license. I was terrified and frustrated all the time.

My medical director at the ER hospital once scolded me after a technician told him how "Dr. K flipped out when she found out we were out of xyz medication." He said to me, "I don't flip out when we're out of something. I consider it an opportunity to think outside the box. I kind of enjoy it, and you should try to look at it that way too." Four years later, his words have finally sunk in.

Now I know that the art of practicing small animal medicine in the real world is the art of improvising. Rolling with the punches and creatively making do with what you've got is what veterinary medicine is really about. That's always what it's been about. It just took me several years of practicing in a variety of different hospitals alongside many other veterinarians before I could finally let go of the medical mirage that I had to practice Gold Standard Veterinary Medicine on every patient, no matter what.

The joy of feeling like you're a good doctor doesn't come from following a recipe out of a cookbook. It comes from remaining flexible and nimble in your thinking despite all kinds of obstacles and limitations, of expertly juggling multiple, conflicting demands in an ever changing environment. It comes from thinking up clever and uniquely appropriate solutions to an endless variety of challenges. It comes from seeing yourself get better every day at creatively making do.

So why don't they teach you how to improvise in vet school? They can't. According to the author of an article in the April 20, 2015 *International Journal of Music Education*, "*True* [sic] improvisation cannot be taught – it is a disposition to be enabled and nurtured."[9] Whether we're talking about the art of medicine or music or painting, the best any educational curriculum can do is to "stimulate the disposition to think creatively."[9] Perhaps someday veterinary schools will offer a course entitled "Medical Improvisation: How to Make the Best with What You've Got," where students will have the opportunity to practice medical improvisation within constraints that mimic the real world. But as it stands today, this is a skill you're just going to have to cultivate on your own when you start practicing. The best recommendation I can offer here is while you're in vet school learning Gold Standard Veterinary Medicine, try to ask yourself questions like, 'What would I do on this case if I could only run one test? What would I do if the client only had $150? Or less? What would I do if the x-ray machine wasn't working or my hospital didn't have an ultrasound machine?'

The ability to medically improvise requires both the knowledge you gained in school and what you learn after school along with a comfortable familiarity with the resources at your disposal. You must combine these in creative yet sensible ways depending on the client and patient you're dealing with. I can't coach you to develop this skill in the span of this book any more than vet school can under their present curricular constrictions.

Becoming good at medical improvisation is a process that takes time and practice. The advantage you have now is you'll be less likely to "flip out" in your first years of practice. Instead, you'll remember to savor the joy of creatively making do.

Papaya #2: Veterinary Medicine is Like Human Medicine, Except the Patients Are Cuter

As I stepped into an education in the hard sciences to qualify for veterinary school, I was enraptured to find myself in a universe where every sliver of knowledge gained was compatible with every other, across the disciplines of mathematics, physics, chemistry, and biology. Mathematics and physics explained and predicted chemical reactions, and chemical reactions explained biology. For the first time in my life - life made sense.

In my application for veterinary school, I wrote in my personal statement: "I want to know what is known, and then I want to know what is not known, and I want to go there to press against that void with every critical thinking, problem solving, intuitive tool at my disposal." I had become a knowledge addict. Studying math and science excited my analytical mind as if I'd applied cocaine directly to my optic nerve. I wanted to know more. I needed to know more. I wanted to race to the edge of everything I'd learned and throw myself over that cliff, happy to fall forever.

When I began studying medicine, I gained molecular, mechanistic understanding of diseases such as rheumatoid arthritis and immune mediated hemolytic anemia, leukemia and lymphoma, diabetes and hypothyroidism. Hungry to comprehend every molecular explanation for the diseases we were learning about, I spent what little free time I had as a veterinary student scouring academic journal articles and every medical textbook that I could get my hands on. Most of the supplemental learning I sought came from human medical literature. The information from those sources was more robust than what I could find in the veterinary medical literature, and I was on a mission to deeply understand every fascinating pathology my professors talked about.

I'd never much enjoyed riddles or brain teasers but in veterinary school I discovered that the application of scientific knowledge to diagnose and treat disease was a puzzle that thrilled like me no other. The idea of being infused with all this medical knowledge and then being able to exercise all my mental faculties to solve medical mysteries and cure my patients was what I looked forward to most in my future career as a veterinarian.

My brain would perform dazzling acrobatic stunts, lithely executing scissor leaps into beranl flips through all the existing medical literature until landing in a perfect arabesque on the right diagnosis. After that, a simple cartwheel would lead to appropriate treatment and my patient would be healed. Of all the veterinary medical mirages I've stepped into only to have them dissipate like water vapor in a desert, this one probably disappointed me the most.

While I think my roving medical curiosity made me a better doctor, knowing how various pathologies are understood, diagnosed and treated in humans became a source of frustration and even sadness when I began practicing. In addition to the limitations of hospital resources and client finances, I also found that less is known about many pathologies in veterinary medicine because the majority of available research dollars are dedicated to advancing human medicine instead.

So for a veterinarian, the thrill of applying scientific knowledge to diagnose and treat disease occurs only in patients who have diseases that are relatively well understood in the veterinary literature. This isn't to say our jobs are easy. Coming to a correct diagnosis of any disease is plenty challenging. It's just that small animal veterinarians outside of academia don't often get to tread beyond the boundaries of the common or the well described. Despite all my longing, as a small animal veterinarian, it isn't for me to press against the void of the unknown.

I've seen many perplexing medical cases that I longed to solve but couldn't. After a particularly frustrating overnight ER shift where the majority of patients remained medical mysteries, despite their owners authorizing me to run every diagnostic test at my disposal, I asked Alex, "Do you ever *not* find out what's wrong with someone in human medicine?" His answer: "Not really. We almost always find out."

I remember him telling me about a patient he saw as a resident in Illinois. The patient had a history of recurrent angioedema - the patient would get swelling in his face and airway - like an allergic reaction. Except this patient did not respond to antihistamines, glucocorticoid steroids or epinephrine injections, as would be expected of someone having an allergic reaction. They had to intubate him to keep his airway open while they sought answers. The doctors hypothesized the patient had a rare disease called hereditary angioedema, the most common variant being a deficiency of the enzyme called c1 esterase inhibitor. This enzyme inhibits spontaneous activation of part of the body's immune system that causes inflammation. They have tests to measure not only the quantity but even the functionality of this enzyme in human medicine. The tests they ran confirmed the diagnosis, and the patient recovered after being treated with concentrated c1 esterase inhibitor. This concentrate can be isolated and harvested from donated blood.

I had never heard of this disorder, had never heard of testing for c1 esterase inhibitor in dogs and cats, nor of concentrated c1 esterase inhibitor being available for veterinary patients. If Alex's patient had been a dog or a cat, he would never have been correctly diagnosed, and he couldn't have been correctly treated. He would either die or be euthanized, becoming just another medical mystery in the life of some sad and frustrated veterinarian. In the six years I've known Alex, he's only confronted one medical mystery that went unsolved. In my five years of practice, one medical mystery was solved.

One night a woman brought in a sweet, little, black Pomeranian named Rhoda to the ER. Rhoda had what appeared to be a mild ear infection. Rhoda's owner told me she didn't want to treat the ear infection. She wanted to euthanize Rhoda. I was horrified. Euthanize a dog for an ear infection? I couldn't do that. "She ain't right," Rhoda's owner said to me as if to rationalize her decision. "She ain't never been right since she was born."

Since I could find no other abnormalities on Rhoda's physical exam, I pleaded with Rhoda's owner to relinquish Rhoda to my hospital. It would cost us little to treat her ear infection and then we could find her a new home. A dog as sweet as Rhoda would be easy to re-home, and if we couldn't find a home for her, I would take her myself. I had already fallen in love with her.

Rhoda's owner agreed, and after she left, we cleaned Rhoda's infected ear and instilled some medication. Rhoda allowed us to do this without complaint, wagging her fluffy, curly tail the whole time. For the duration of my shift, whenever I sat at my desk to type medical records or review test results on other patients, Rhoda sat happily in my lap. She lovingly licked my chin every time I gazed down at her. After doctors' rounds the next morning, I drove home feeling happy that I had been able to save such a sweet dog. I was off duty for the next two days but planned on checking in by phone to see how Rhoda was doing.

Rhoda's health completely unraveled during the course of those two days. First she developed intractable vomiting and diarrhea. Blood work and x-rays did not provide any answers. Then she developed a head tilt. Then she developed heart failure, severe pulmonary edema and respiratory distress. The Internal Medicine doctor at my hospital wasn't even able to figure out what was wrong with her. I spoke with my medical director and agreed with sadness that Rhoda should be euthanized. She was suffering, and since we didn't know what was wrong with her, we didn't know how to help her.

How could so many things go so wrong in such a short span of time in a patient that initially presented for a simple ear infection? I racked my brain for plausible explanations. I scoured the Veterinary Information Network (VIN) online. I talked to Alex about Rhoda's case. It was of no use. There were plenty of clues but little evidence. Without exhaustive diagnostic tests, there was no way to arrive at a definitive answer.

Because my hospital had a small fund for doctors to run tests for their own education, I asked my medical director to send Rhoda's body to a pathologist for a necropsy (in human medicine this procedure is called an autopsy). I received the pathologist's report a week later. The pathologist had found abnormal nerve fibers in multiple organ systems throughout Rhoda's body. The diagnosis was something I'd never learned about in veterinary school: Neurofibromatosis. It's a genetically inherited disease that causes abnormal growth and invasion of nerve fibers into various tissues and organs in the body. These abnormal nerve fibers can cause malfunction in any of the infiltrated organs.

In the first twenty-five results returned from my search for Neurofibromatosis on VIN, all of them were from human medical or human research journals except for one article in a journal called *Lab Animal* and one vet-to-vet discussion that turned out to be more about a different condition (fibrosarcoma) with one veterinarian merely mentioning he'd heard of neurofibromatosis.

If Rhoda had been a human, she likely would have seen multiple specialists, had CT scans, MRIs, biopsies with histopathology, and genetic testing in order to get her diagnosis. The most likely treatment for her would have been an attempted surgical resection of the aberrant nerve fibers. Even for an MD surgical specialist this would be a difficult procedure because the nerve fibers can be tiny and very closely associated with, and adhered to, other anatomical structures. Additionally, there would be no guarantee the operation would be successful in alleviating her symptoms. Even if it were, the underlying genetic abnormality would not be cured and she would likely suffer more symptoms in the future from ongoing infiltration of these aberrant nerve fibers into various body systems. Still, had Rhoda been a human, she would have gotten this operation, as well as subsequent operations if they had the potential of improving and extending her life.

There are numerous charities raising money to fund medical research for neurofibromatosis in humans. While I don't know how likely this research is to yield improved treatment options or even a cure for people with this condition in the foreseeable future, I do know the chances of this happening for non-human animals with neurofibromatosis are about as good as the chances that teleportation will become available in my lifetime.

Rhoda's case gave me a glimpse into a world I will never set foot in. A world where doctors make every attempt and spare no expense to figure out what's going on with a patient, a world where they "almost always" figure it out, and a world where fixing the patient remains the ultimate objective even at the cost of tens of thousands or sometimes even hundreds of thousands of dollars. Despite all my passion for medicine and my insatiable hunger for ever increasing medical knowledge, as a veterinarian, that is the kind of doctor I can never be.

Disheartening as this realization was, it taught me an invaluable lesson. It put into perspective every subsequent medical mystery I've since encountered. A medical condition that is not discoverable through the the diagnostic tests available to veterinarians is also not likely to be curable using the available treatment protocols. And if the cure to a medical mystery doesn't exist in veterinary medicine, the educational value of solving that mystery is negligible to me as a small animal veterinarian. I couldn't have saved Rhoda's life even if I'd been able to figure out what was wrong with her.

So, I no longer obsess over medical mysteries, wasting time pouring over medical literature in search of answers I will either never find or that will do my patients no good. Because of what I learned from Rhoda, instead of banging my head against the void of the unknown, I am at peace with my limitations as a veterinarian. I am resigned to the fact that veterinary medicine is not just like human medicine. There will be many things I can't figure out, and many patients I can't fix, because there are many things we just don't know.

Apple #2: The crabgrass on the other side

It's true I envy my husband's superior training and medical knowledge, the seemingly limitless diagnostic options he has at his disposal, the battalion of medical specialists he has to call upon for help, the medical mysteries he gets to solve, but that being said, I'm still glad I became a DVM instead of an MD, and here are two reasons why.

Patients who refuse to be fixed - and are not cute

If an owner brings her diabetic cat to me for a recheck and I run some tests that indicate the cat's diabetes has not been well controlled, or an owner of a dog with severe allergies brings her dog back to me after being MIA for several months and the dog is now covered head to toe in red, scabby crusts and clearly needed to see me sooner, or if a patient returns the day after a laceration repair having chewed her sutures out because the owner didn't follow my instructions to keep the Elizabethan collar on... I don't blame my patients. None of this is their fault. I still love them, and my desire to help them is undiminished. As a veterinarian, all my patients really are cute, become they are all blameless.

My father was 5'2" and weighed 230 pounds. He had uncontrolled diabetes. He was on two different types of insulin. He was to inject himself with 44 units of Lantus insulin twice a day, and 15 units of Humalog insulin three times a day. He was prescribed multiple oral medications for the various complications he'd developed due to his unwillingness to properly manage his diabetes. He refused to check his blood sugar regularly because he didn't want to waste glucometer needles. He refused to take his oral medications as prescribed because of the side effects he'd read about. He did not use his injectable insulin as directed. He repeatedly told me he was going to reverse his diabetes through dieting but his freezer was full of ice cream and his cupboards contained dozens of boxes of macaroni and cheese and sugary breakfast cereals. I spoke with his GP before he passed away. She told me the last time he visited her for a checkup he informed her she was mismanaging his diabetes because he read on the internet that insulin is poisonous.

Imagine being a human medical doctor and having to deal with patients like my father. His non-compliance was extreme, but not unique. How many people do you know who have medical issues but refuse to follow their doctor's orders? Perhaps you know someone with heart disease who continues to eat fatty, high-salt foods? How many people actually lose weight because their doctor told them to? Or stop smoking or drinking because their doctor told them to? Or even take their medications like they're supposed to? Imagine having the most extensive arsenal of medical knowledge, diagnostic and treatment options available only to find yourself unable to fix many your patients because they refuse to be fixed.

I don't know about you, but I think I might find that even more demoralizing than not being able to figure out what's wrong with every one of my patients. I would not find patients like my father cute at all! I like to love my patients, even the mean ones. As a veterinarian, I can, because whatever it is that's wrong with them - it's not their fault. It's never their fault.

The catch-22 of patients who can't be fixed

If a geriatric miniature poodle in excruciating pain, covered in blood, and struggling to breathe after being attacked by a coyote presents as an emergency walk-in, and I learn this poodle belongs to an elderly lady who already has her hands full taking care of her husband who's dying of lung cancer, or if I see a twelve year old, white-muzzled Labrador retriever who started having seizures a month ago and is now pressing his head against walls and refusing to eat, or an eighteen year old cat with chronic kidney disease who is no longer responding to therapy, I have the power to save these patients and their owners from the horrors that a prolonged, natural death can bring. I have the power to end suffering in an instant.

Despite the miracles of modern medicine, sometimes human medical doctors don't figure out what's wrong until it's too late to fix. Also, they can't reverse aging or the systemic damage caused by chronic illness. Eventually, even the healthiest bodies degenerate beyond their ability to repair. What happens when human medical doctors can't fix what's wrong?

When I got the call at 5AM from my father's cellular number, but the voice on the line was not my father's, I knew something terrible had happened. "It was a stroke," the medical resident explained to me, "a massive stroke. Your father is unable to move, speak or swallow." I was on a plane to Chicago the next day. My father was still alert and aware when I arrived. He could move his eyes and look around. He could nod and shake his head slowly to answer yes or no. But that was all. A CT scan revealed a severe pontine stroke. Medically, nothing could be done to reverse the damage and restore functionality.

There were still options though. Even though he couldn't eat, I knew they could place a stomach tube so food could be pumped into his gastrointestinal tract. Even though his inability to swallow caused saliva and mucous to accumulate in the back of this throat, making it difficult for him to breathe, I knew they could place a tube through his neck directly into his airway to make breathing easler. I knew he could be transferred to a long-term care facility where nurse's aids would change his diapers and bathe and dress him every day. They would turn him every few hours to avoid bed sores. He could vegetate like that until the next medical problem brought him back to the hospital, and they would patch him up and send him out again. And again. And again.

Even before I arrived at the hospital, before I'd talked to any of the attending physicians, the hospital social workers were calling me. They called me before I boarded the flight to Phoenix. They called me while I was waiting for my connecting flight to Chicago. They wanted me to make a decision. They wanted my father out of the hospital - either to long-term care or home to die.

I knew I couldn't care my father at home. He was too heavy for me to be able to keep him clean and comfortable as he waited for death. I also suspected my father wouldn't want to go to a long term-care facility. He had repeatedly told me he would rather die than go to a nursing home. I resisted the pressure from the social workers until I could speak face to face with the hospital doctors. From them, I learned that my father could be admitted to in-hospital hospice, which would save him the discomfort and indignity of being moved in his present state. This service was reserved only for people not expected to live more than a week. If I authorized withdrawal of fluid therapy, my father would be unlikely to survive that long.

I explained the situation as gently as I could to my father. "I'm so sorry, but they can't fix what's happened to you, Dad. You're not going to recover the ability to move, or speak or swallow. We can move you to long-term care, but they would need to place a stomach tube and a breathing tube." He shook his head. A tear from his left eye streamed down the side of his face onto the perfectly white hospital pillow. He'd made his decision. I asked the doctors to stop the IV fluids.

He was permitted "comfort feedings." If the objective were to keep him alive this wouldn't have been an option because it would increase his chances of developing pneumonia. But since the goal instead was to keep him as comfortable as possible until he died, the nurses brought trays of cherry Jell-O, yogurt, soup broth, and coffee. I spooned Jell-O and yogurt into his mouth, and I dipped a small sponge on a stick into the broth and coffee and pressed the sponge against the inside of his cheek to release the liquid in his mouth. He was only able to successfully swallow a quarter of the time. The rest of the time, the soft foods and liquids either spilled out of his mouth and down his chin or entered his airway causing him to choke and cough. Once a day a hospice nurse came to bathe him and change his sheets.

The doctors started him on a morphine constant rate infusion to reduce his discomfort. Pneumonia would inevitably develop as bacteria-ridden food and saliva entered his airway and lungs. Pneumonia makes breathing more and more difficult as it worsens. I've heard it said that nothing is worse than "air hunger." The morphine dose would be increased as my father's air hunger increased.

On the third day of this ordeal, as I was sponging coffee with cream and sugar into his mouth, I said to him, "Dad, I'm going to ask you one more time." His eyes fixed on mine, fully attentive. "Do you want to change your mind? Do you want a stomach tube placed?" He shook his head, "No." "Am I doing the right thing for you?" He nodded his head, "Yes." It was two more days before he slipped into unconsciousness, and another twelve hours after that before he died. Those five and a half miserable days of waiting for death was the best human medicine could do for him.

I've experienced the other side of the spectrum too. It's much worse. My mother became very ill when I was a second year veterinary student. At that juncture in my education, I still thought the television show *House, MD* was a realistic depiction of modern medicine. Because of my ignorance, my mother spent the last months of her life on a ventilator. I'm just thankful they never performed CPR on her. That certainly would have broken her ribs, and because of the severe osteoporosis she'd developed from the steroids she'd been on for years, CPR probably would have broken her spine as well.

I would give anything to be able to go back in time and make a different choice for her. I would exchange all the remaining years of my own life for the chance to spoon feed her yogurt and Jell-O for five miserable days rather than letting her suffer for months and die alone on a ventilator because I thought there was some small chance she might recover, and none of the doctors could convince this naive second year veterinary student otherwise.

For all the incredible things human medicine can do, in the United States, except for physicians in a handful of states, human medical doctors frequently face the catch-22 of having to either let their terminally ill patients die slowly and naturally, or of having to prolong their lives unnaturally when family members can't be made to understand the horrors of what they're demanding. No, thank you. If I didn't have the power to the end needless suffering, I don't think I could practice medicine at all.

16 Things I Learned the Hard Way

"Learn from the mistakes of others. You can't live long enough to make them all yourself."
- Eleanor Roosevelt

1. **Listen to your gut.** As you go about your busy day as a small animal veterinarian, your inner dialogue will chatter incessantly. Loudest and hardest to ignore will be the negative backseat driver I told you about in Book 1. That's the voice you want to argue with rather than passively believing. But there is another voice. A much quieter voice. A voice that hates to intrude and only does so when it has something important to say. I don't know which part of the brain this quiet voice comes from. I don't know if it comes from the brain at all. Maybe it comes from the neural plexus in the GI tract, the gut. Maybe it comes from God, or guardian angels, or Native

American Animal Spirits.

Wherever it comes from, it always urges caution, and it's always right. Every time I've ignored it, the knapsack of regret I carry around with me has grown heavier. This quiet voice says things like, "ignore everyone and everything else going on right now - do not rush through this" or "this is one of those times when you need to go by the book" or "there is something besides the obvious going on here" or "take a deep breath, steady your mind and try again" or "even though that dog is wagging his tail, don't trust him."

When I hear this voice it's as if someone tapped a crystal glass inside my head. The message rises above the din of all the other self-talk with a high-pitched, rich tone that resonates for just a moment. It's unambiguous, to the point, and never repeated. I'm not sure if you'll experience this voice the same way so you need to pay attention and learn how to recognize it in your own head. Heed its counsel no matter what else is going on. It always seems to speak to me at the most inconvenient times - when there is a tornado of activity causing technicians, office managers, clients, other patients, telephones, hospital equipment, and sometimes even other veterinarians to fly through the air in distracting circles around me – which is why it's so tempting to ignore it. Don't.

New doctors are especially prone to ignoring this voice. New doctors feel like they should be able to handle everything without hesitating or showing doubt. They fear they'll be criticized for over-reacting if they slow down, or do more than what seems necessary, or are overly cautious, or ask for guidance. Experienced doctors don't worry about appearing hesitant, or asking for help, or being criticized for slowing down - because they've learned the hard way that it's always better to err on the side of caution than to ignore that quiet voice and suffer the guilt and shame of a bad outcome later.

2. **Establish your medical boundaries.** It's really hard to do this when you're just starting out. You're going to feel pulled in so many different directions. Should you do xyz the way your professors told you to? Should you do it the way the technicians tell you it's done at this hospital? Should you do it the way your boss wants you to do it? There are dozens of possible ways to do everything - from performing exams and taking histories to placing IV catheters and doing surgery.

   After I left emergency medicine, I started working at what must be the worst day practice ever to exist on the planet. Still keenly aware of my own inexperience however, I didn't want to appear dogmatic or rigid so I tried to keep an open mind. I went with the flow and regretted it. No one told me this before I started practicing, but the worst kind of regret is the kind that comes from facing a poor medical outcome because you practiced the way someone else told you to.

Because of the tremendous variability of resources and standards of care in veterinary medicine, part of the burden of responsibility that comes with being a veterinarian is mustering the courage to stand firm on your own principles of practice. You must decide for yourself what you will and won't do, how you will and won't do things, and under what circumstances. The medical boundaries you develop will have to take into account economic factors in addition to your own medical judgment. For example, shelters and low-cost spay/neuter clinics may operate on such tight budgets that the added costs of a higher standard of care would reduce the number of animals they are able to help. You may trespass against your own medical boundaries on a case dependent basis. Perhaps in some cases you'll have to choose between your medical boundaries and helping an animal at all. Your boundaries may change as you gain experience. However, these are choices for *you* to make as the doctor. They're not for someone else to impose upon you against your better judgment.

Since you're accountable for the consequences, you're responsible for establishing your own medical boundaries and for defending them despite any pressure you may face from support staff, other veterinarians or pet owners. It won't be easy. It will take time for you to even figure out what your own medical boundaries are, and under what conditions you're willing to violate them. Then it will take intestinal fortitude to fight for your right to practice according to your own standards. But it is your right - and your responsibility - as a doctor. Don't let anyone try to convince you otherwise. Following are my top six medical boundaries. You can use them as a guide before you develop your own, or reject them. The choice is yours.

I perform a proper scrub and wear a gown, cap, mask, and gloves for every surgery, and every surgical patient gets his own, sterile surgery pack, and a brand new scalpel blade. This is proper aseptic surgical technique. To save time or money, some hospitals don't practice proper aseptic surgical technique. The owner of the worst day practice ever told me that dogs and cats have different bacterial flora than humans, therefore we didn't have to use aseptic surgical protocols. Then one of his patients developed septic peritonitis after a cryptorchid surgery.

Every patient undergoing surgery has an IV catheter placed and is on IV fluids during surgery, except in rare cases where fluids are contraindicated. Some hospitals balk at this because it increases the cost of surgery and the cost to clients. But the actual cost of a catheter, a fluid line and a bag of fluids is only about $30. I include these costs in my estimates and explain to clients why an IV catheter and IV fluids during surgery are necessary. Every cell and organ in the body needs oxygen. Blood carries oxygen. Blood flow depends on blood pressure. Anesthesia causes blood pressure to drop. IV fluids keep blood pressure normalized, reduce stress on the heart and protect the kidneys.

The kidneys are extremely sensitive to low blood flow and can be easily damaged if their blood supply is restricted, even for short periods. Think of a garden hose. If you turn the faucet down you reduce water pressure and less water comes out. It's the same with the blood vessels throughout the body including those feeding the kidneys. Anesthesia turns the faucet down. IV fluids turn the faucet back up.

I once saw a very good veterinarian perform a routine surgery on a cat who was not on IV fluids. This particular hospital didn't routinely give IV fluids to patients under anesthesia and this vet was simply going with the flow. After the cat recovered, the vet realized she had forgotten to check the pre-operative blood work on the cat. This is easy to do in a busy clinic when you're juggling many things at once. I too have forgotten to check pre-operative blood work before starting a surgery – I was just lucky the blood work was normal.

This vet wasn't so lucky. It turned out this healthy appearing cat had kidney disease. Being under anesthesia without IV fluids worsened the cat's kidney disease and likely shaved years off her life. I don't tell you this story to criticize this other veterinarian. There but for the grace of God go I. I tell this story to impress upon you the dramatic drop in blood pressure that can occur under anesthesia and the damage it can cause. Healthy animals may be better able to tolerate this, they may be better able to recover afterwards but I can't say their chances of developing kidney disease don't increase after an insult like this.

Of more immediate medical concern is the heart. The heart has to pump harder and faster when an animal is under anesthesia because it's trying to turn the faucet back up to maintain blood flow throughout the body, including to the kidneys. When the heart has to work harder it requires more blood and oxygen for itself. If the heart is unable to turn the faucet up enough, it doesn't get the blood flow it needs either, and cardiac arrest can occur. IV fluids turn the faucet up so the heart doesn't have to work so hard.

Lastly, in the event a pet does suffer cardiac arrest under anesthesia, having an IV catheter in place with fluids already running means the doctor can push emergency drugs into the patient immediately, and the chances of a successful resuscitation increase. Placing an IV catheter after an animal's heart has stopped is much more difficult and sometimes impossible. If an IV catheter isn't already in place when an animal suffers an arrest, the chances for successful resuscitation decrease drastically.

Elective dental surgeries are limited to two hours or less. I created this medical boundary after losing a patient during a dental. The patient had such terrible dental disease she needed almost all of her teeth extracted. Accomplishing this would have taken four hours. She died at two and a half hours. We were unable to resuscitate her. Her name was Saturn. She was sweet and gentle, and I carry her memory - and the memory of her incredibly kind and understanding owners - in my broken heart every day.

Since then, I tell owners whose pets have severe dental disease that, for their pet's safety, I will not keep their pet under anesthesia longer than two hours. If we cannot finish during that time, another procedure will have to be scheduled, even though it will be more costly. Owners have been invariably cooperative when I explained that the risk of complications under anesthesia, including death, increase after two hours. Sometimes we have to take that risk, such as for some emergency surgeries, or even elective orthopedic surgeries like total hip replacements or tibial plateau leveling osteotomies. But we don't have to take that risk for an elective dental surgery.

No ovariohysterectomies on dogs over 30 pounds who are in heat, or pregnant (well, maybe if they're pregnant). In both cases, the blood vessels leading to and from the reproductive tract are engorged and enormous.
The bigger the blood vessels, the more difficult it is to tie them off and the greater the chances of potentially fatal internal bleeding. The tissues of dogs in estrus are also more fragile in general. If I find a dog to be in heat on examination, I tell the owners we can schedule the surgery in 4 weeks, after she's come out of estrus. If a c-section is needed on a pregnant dog, this is a more difficult decision.

We can open the uterus, remove the babies, close the uterus, and complete the surgery without spaying the dog, or we can remove the babies, and then perform an ovariohysterectomy. Most vets prefer the latter, because it eliminates the chances of another pregnancy, future pyometra (uterine infection), and further exacerbation of the problem of pet over-population. Ultimately, the choice is up to the pet owner. Breeders often do not want an ovariohysterectomy because they want to breed the dog again. This makes the decision simple.

What about owners who have no plans to breed the dog again? It's certainly safer to just take out the puppies and not perform a spay because of those enormous blood vessels feeding the reproductive tract. However, if we don't perform the spay during this surgery, the owners will have to pay for another surgery later. If I explain the risks to the owners and they tell me they're fine with scheduling a spay later, that's fantastic. But what if the owners aren't able or willing to pay for another surgery later?

Then I have to make sure they understand the higher risk of potentially fatal internal bleeding. I also have to insist that after the surgery, the dog remains in the hospital for monitoring until I feel she's safe to go home. This isn't ideal for her puppies. Their baby immune systems are especially vulnerable to infectious diseases, but they need to nurse, so they need to stay with momma.

Additionally, since c-sections tend to be emergency surgeries, we may be nearing closing time by the time I finish the surgery. Momma dog can't stay overnight in the hospital unattended. She needs to go to the local ER for overnight monitoring. The cost of overnight hospitalization at an ER could easily be more than what the cost of a spay would have been. What if the owners can't afford it? This is why the question of whether or not to perform an ovario-hysterectomy in a pregnant dog can be difficult. I worry less about little dogs with smaller blood vessels, but much more about bigger dogs with bigger blood vessels.

I use good pain control protocols for my surgeries, and post-operative patients get sent home with pain medications. No, I will not perform surgery on your pet and not send home pain medications just so you can save a few bucks. At the last hospital I worked, we solved the problem of pet owners wanting to save money by declining post-operative pain medications by simply including the pain medications in the total cost of the surgery. We did the same thing with IV fluids. If it's not a line item on the estimate, it's not up for negotiation. Problem solved: The pet gets good medical care, and the doctors get peace of mind.

No examinations, vaccinations, nail trims, ear cleanings or anything else on aggressive animals without sedation. I won't risk the safety of my staff or myself just to save time or so a pet owner doesn't have to spend money on sedating their aggressive pet. A single bite to one of my hands – even from a cat - has the potential to end my career. It's happened to other people, and they've required hand surgery after hand surgery, and still didn't get full functionality restored.

I am not dissuaded from this stance no matter how upset a client gets or how much they argue. Nope, no way, heck no. Furthermore, attempting to restrain an aggressive animal only fuels their distrust and hatred of veterinary hospitals and personnel. I'm not talking about sedating every pet that looks at me sideways. For patients who are merely wary, a muzzle will usually do (and this too is non-negotiable). I'm talking about the animals that are so aggressive they will literally try to kill you if you touch them.

3. **You need silence, and it's okay to ask for it.** There are four stages of learning.[11] We begin as *unconsciously incompetent*, meaning we don't know and we don't even know we don't know. Ignorance is bliss. This is where the "bright-eyed graduating medical student" first steps onto the stage as a shiny, new and enthusiastic veterinarian – "bursting with altruism" and "full of dreams."[10] The next stage is *conscious incompetence*, where we still don't know, but now we know we don't know. Ouch. This is the most unpleasant of the four stages. We are slow, awkward, often wrong, and frustrated during this stage. After conscious incompetence, we progress to *consciously competent*. Finally, we're getting good at

what we do – but we're still slow because we need to think very carefully about everything. At last, we ascend to *unconscious competence*. This is the sweet spot where things just seem to come naturally. We know our jobs so well we hardly need to think about it at all. When we reach this stage we can relax and have a little fun.

After you outgrow the initial bliss of being a new veterinarian and progress to the consciously incompetent and consciously competent stages of learning, you will find the casual conversations of technicians and other support staff maddeningly distracting. I did. I would be trying to reason my way through a complex medical case or trying to perform a surgery or some kind of procedure, even a simple laceration repair, and the people around me would be talking about their favorite bands, or their boyfriends, or clothes, or whatever. Secretly, I wanted to scream, "SHUT UP! Can't you see I'm trying to do something important here?!" Of course, I would never say that out loud. I simply fumed with anger and resentment in complete silence. But the support staff weren't being intentionally inconsiderate. They were used to working with experienced veterinarians.

After I started moving into the unconsciously competent stage, I realized that the talking of the support staff around me no longer impeded my ability to think or perform. Now I know it's completely normal to need silence when you're a new vet. So instead of getting silently upset like I did, just ask for the silence you need. All you have to say is, "Hey guys, I'm sorry to have to ask this of you, but since I'm inexperienced, what I'm doing (or thinking about) right now is pretty difficult and I really need some quiet, please. Thank you so much." You can say this later in your career too any time you're tackling something difficult. Just don't forget to tell them when it's okay to start talking again;)

4. **You set the pace.** As you're scrutinizing the abdominal radiographs of a sick patient you're very concerned about, one of your technicians will have a question about pet food from a client she's speaking with on the phone. Another technician will need you to fill out a prescription for a post-operative patient who's being discharged. The front desk receptionist will ask if she can add another appointment to your already fully booked schedule. Your veterinary assistant will tell you that the clients in exam room two are waiting to talk to you and also that she was not able to get blood for the heartworm test you ordered. Your office manager will need to speak with you about the client who complained that you didn't examine her cat's ears when she brought him in for his annual appointment.

   In the eye of storms like this, which occur every day in the working life of a veterinarian, lies your next medical error. Support staff and clients don't know what's going through your mind or how hard you're thinking. They have their own reasons for hurrying you or wanting you to do something in the moment, but you are the doctor, and you set the pace. If you need things to slow down, if you need to make a client wait, if you need to not take that telephone call or answer your technician's question because something else is more important – so be it. Take a deep breath, and inform them how much time you need before you can do what they want you to do. Be polite about it, but don't ever allow anyone to rush you.

5. **Round with your support staff before every shift.** "Medical rounds," sometimes just called "rounds," are typically where doctors and/or support staff discuss patients' problems, tests and test results, diagnoses, treatments, progress, and prognosis. The point of medical rounds is usually to bring staff coming on shift up to speed (such as in a 24-hour emergency hospital). The emergency hospital where I worked had separate medical rounds for doctors and technicians. The doctor finishing a shift updated the doctor starting a shift. Ditto for technicians. The first time I witnessed medical rounds at a day practice was at the last (and the best) place I worked. It was not a 24-hour hospital so the purpose of medical rounds was different. The medical rounds at this day practice consisted of doctors and support staff discussing together all scheduled appointments

for the day in order to formulate an organized, coordinated plan.

For example, say the 1 o'clock appointment is for a young dog with diarrhea. Your team can decide in advance that the dog should be checked for intestinal worms, and you can have one of your support staff call the owner ahead of time and instruct her to bring a stool sample to the appointment. As soon as the owner arrives, one of the support staff can begin processing the stool sample and performing the fecal analysis. Before you even perform your examination you may already know the dog is positive for hookworms and roundworms.

Say the 2 o'clock appointment is for what the owner described as a "big, red, painful bump next to the anus." Sounds like an anal gland abscess that needs to be lanced and drained. Though it's a simple procedure, because of the required sedation, it can be time consuming. Luckily, the 2:30 appointment slot is open. You and your support staff agree to block it off to ensure adequate time to perform the procedure. Does this mean everyone needs to arrive 15 minutes early in the morning to round before appointments begin? Yes. But it also means the day will go more smoothly and you'll all be less likely to have to stay late.

One of my surgery professors in veterinary school, and the only professor in the teaching hospital who seemed to have any semblance of a work-life balance, was fond of saying, "Control the controllable." Whether you end up working in ER, specialty or day practice, rounding with your support staff before every shift to plan ahead is the best way I know of doing this. Doctors' days are filled with unpredictability. Your best hope for coping gracefully with the uncontrollable is to control the controllable.

In an ER, of course, there is no set schedule. No one can predict what kind of medical emergency will walk in the door. But you and your team can decide in advance things like who's going to be responsible for caring for the hospitalized patients versus helping with outpatient care, or who's going to take care of patients in the isolation room. You can also brief your team on things like which hospitalized patient you're most concerned about and what you want your support staff to watch for.

6. **Don't try to solve every case.** When I worked in the ER and someone brought in a happy, tail-wagging dog with diarrhea in the middle of the night who was otherwise normal on physical exam, I didn't feel bad about not coming to a definitive diagnosis for the diarrhea. I had critically ill patients in the hospital and life threatening emergencies being carried through the front door who needed my time and attention much more. When I transitioned to day practice though, I thought it was my job to solve every case I encountered. After all, I was the GP. If the buck didn't stop with me, then who did it stop with?

This may not be the most important medical tip I can give you, but it's the one most likely to preserve your sanity if you decide to be a general practice veterinarian. Don't think you need to solve every case you see. First of all, it's impossible. Most days, there will simply not be enough time in your schedule to do a deep dive into every single case. Second of all, it's unnecessary. Most of the patients you'll see with mild signs of illness will get better with symptomatic treatment (treatments targeted at the symptoms rather than the underlying cause of the symptoms) or empirical treatment (treatment based on your medically educated guess as to what the underlying cause might be). Thirdly, if you try to solve every case you see, the *really* sick patients who *really* need you will suffer the consequences of your diluted attention, energy and time. Fourthly, if you try to solve every case you will exasperate your coworkers and burn yourself out.

So here's how to not solve a case. First establish the pet is stable. "Stable" means the pet is acting relatively normal, is eating, drinking, urinating and defecating normally, and your physical exam findings are unimpressive. The pet does not require hospitalization, is not in eminent danger of dying, and is not experiencing pain severe enough to require IV pain medications. Consider best and worst case scenarios that may explain the signs that prompted the owners to bring the pet in. Communicate these with the owners. Tell the owners you are going to provide symptomatic or empirical treatment based on the best case scenario – but you could be wrong. Make it very clear to the owners that if the pet does not get better or if he gets worse he must be re-evaluated by a doctor. Then implement the treatment, write the prescription and move on.

Is it possible there will be something more serious going on and you'll miss it? Always. This is why you must impress upon the owners the importance of having their pet re-examined if he doesn't get better. If the pet is stable when he sees you, his health is unlikely to decline so precipitously that intervention at a later time won't provide a successful remedy. Illness is dynamic, and often, even if a patient is developing a serious illness, the signs and symptoms in the early stages may be too subtle to be helpful. Sometimes, even if we want to solve a case, it's necessary for us to wait for the nature of the illness to "declare itself." So, yes. Some small percentage of patients you treat symptomatically or empirically will need further medical attention. This is not a medical failure. It's a fact of medical practice – whether veterinary or human.

I once saw a bright and alert, seven year old black lab who had stopped eating, according to his owners. "He's always hungry," Mrs. Owner said to me, "so when he doesn't want to eat, I know something must be wrong." The dog had no history of eating inappropriate things, was wagging his tail and excitedly gulping down all the dog cookies I offered. His physical exam was normal, he hadn't been vomiting, he had had a bowel movement that morning, and he let me squeeze his belly like he thought it was a wonderful massage. The only reason I did any diagnostic testing at all was because he was very thin. I did blood work to rule out any obvious metabolic disorders that could explain his low body condition score. Maybe he had kidney disease with protein losing nephropathy. That could cause both weight loss and loss of appetite. But his blood work was completely normal.

On further questioning, the owner told me he had lost weight because they put him on a diet! (Forehead slap!) He had been too fat. I asked if they had increased the amount he was fed each day since he lost the weight he needed to lose? No. I did a quick calculation and realized he was being fed too little for a dog his size. I told the owner I didn't know why he didn't eat for her earlier but he sure seemed to have a good appetite here in the exam room. Maybe he just had a transient tummy ache and now he was better. Since his blood work looked great and his physical exam was normal I suggested she take him home and see how he did. I gave her information on how much he needed to be eating every day in order to maintain a healthy weight, and of course, told her to bring him back if he didn't improve or got worse. In my mind, I had actually done a great job on this case.

He got worse though. I was off the next day when the owners brought him back to my hospital. He still wasn't eating and he had started vomiting. Abdominal x-rays were done and he was diagnosed with a gastro-intestinal obstruction. A pillow case was surgically removed from his small intestine. He had probably eaten it because he was starving! When I heard what had happened, I initially felt terrible. I should have done x-rays. But you know what? They could have easily appeared normal because it was too early in the development of the blockage. Or they might have appeared suspicious but not suspicious enough to warrant surgery, in which case, my recommendation would have been the same: Take him home, monitor and bring him back if he doesn't get better. There are plenty of past mistakes I still beat myself up for. This isn't one of them.

7. **It's not your fault every time a patient dies.** I can't remember which of my professors said this but Alex has heard a similar saying from doctors who practice on humans: "50% will get better with standard treatment, 30% will get better no matter what you do, 10% will die no matter what you do, and in only 10% of the cases will your heroics or genius, or lack thereof, mean the difference between life and death." I can't vouch for the accuracy of these percentages but my experience and instincts roughly agree.

The problem in veterinary medicine is that we often don't know for certain what the cause of death was in our patients, so we have a tendency to come up with multiple explanations for how it might have been our fault. Either it was something we did, but shouldn't have, or it was something we didn't do, but should have. It's part of our perfectionist nature. If we made a mistake we want to know so we can be sure to never make that mistake again.

I don't think it's possible, or even completely beneficial, for veterinarians not to question themselves after the death of a patient. I just think we should add one more question to our post-mortem ruminations: Is it possible this animal would have died no matter what we did? Then remember, the answer may be yes.

8. **The worst time to train for an emergency is during an emergency.** I'm talking about CPR, or cardio respiratory resuscitation. ER staff are typically well trained on CPR protocols and procedures, although don't take this for granted. But the day practices where I've worked had no CPR protocols and none of the staff were trained for CPR. Wherever you end up practicing, find out if they have CPR protocols and whether their staff are trained for CPR. If not, create the protocols and conduct the training.

The best role for the doctor to take during CPR is that of director. You should be telling other staff members what role to play, supervising their performance and keeping track of time. You should not be performing chest compressions, intubating, ventilating, placing an IV catheter, or programming the fluid pump to bolus IV fluids. If your support staff aren't trained in advance, you're going to end up having to do things you shouldn't be doing. This means you won't be able to effectively direct, and the chances of saving the patient will decrease.

Make sure CPR training is conducted on a regular basis and that new employees don't get left out of the loop. The last tip I'll offer on this topic really applies to practice in general but is especially critical in emergencies. Never say, "I need someone to xyz…" Always specify exactly *who* is to do *what*. Make eye contact, say their name and give them the task. Do this for every task. When you ask "someone" to do something, it usually ends up getting done by no one.

9. **For sick patients, get the history yourself.** In the ER the technicians were great at getting brief patient histories that included only the information I needed to take the next step. What's the signalment (age, sex, breed)? What's the presenting complaint? What's the patient's TPR (temperature, pulse and respiration), gum color and attitude? For example they might tell me, "Eight year old, female, spayed German shepherd acting lethargic since yesterday. TPR normal. Gum color normal. She's ambulatory, alert and wagging her tail." That's really all a

technician or veterinary assistant should tell me about a sick patient. I need to get the rest of the history myself after performing a physical exam. Only after I examine the patient will I know which questions need to be asked next.

For some reason, in day practice, the technicians would spend half the appointment or more getting a history on a sick patient, and that history often turned out to be either unnecessary or misleading. I think it's partly because day practice support staff are accustomed to seeing mostly wellness visits with healthy pets who are coming in for vaccines and heartworm tests. In those cases it's okay for them to take half the appointment. What the doctor needs to do for those patients is straightforward and takes a limited and pretty predictable amount of time.

Additionally, clients tend to be more talkative when they bring their pets to their "regular" veterinarian, even if their pets are sick. It's hard for support staff to feel comfortable being assertive enough with clients to extricate themselves from the conversation. I think they literally feel trapped in the room sometimes by talkative pet owners who may very well end up feeling slighted by an abrupt technician – something that truly will not do in a general practice where client relationships are what it's all about.

The problem is it's impossible to predict how much of your time a sick patient will need. It's very possible they'll need more than the time allotted for the appointment. Furthermore, the sicker the patient, the more crucial the physical exam becomes, which is an additional reason for you to see sick patients quickly rather than waiting for your support staff to get a history. Lastly, the sicker the patient, the more necessary it becomes to lean toward Gold Standard Veterinary Medicine – and the closer you get to that standard, the more time you will need.

When you're operating on a set schedule, every minute you spend on an appointment beyond the time scheduled means either the next patient has to wait longer or you're going to end up juggling multiple appointments and multiple patients. This dilutes your effectiveness and increases the stress for both you and your support staff. My advice, if you end up as a general practitioner, is ask support staff to put owners with sick pets in an exam room and say, "Mrs. Jones, I understand we think there might be something wrong with Fluffy and I want her to be seen as soon as possible so I'm going to get the doctor now." This phrase is a great tool for support staff to use because it enables them to cut short a conversation with an owner in a way that lets the owner know they are doing it out of concern for the pet. Then go in with your assistant and get the entire history yourself either after or while you're performing the physical exam. Trust me. It will be better for everyone this way.

Another important thing to teach your support

staff if you're a GP is that patients presenting for "wellness visits" or annual exams sometimes turn out to be sick. When that's the case, the doctor may elect not to vaccinate at all and instead implement a completely different algorithm. Therefore I recommend you ask your support staff to stop and come to get you if they observe something concerning or if the owner starts reporting signs of possible illness. All they have to say is, "Mrs. Jones, I'm a little concerned about what you're telling me (or what I'm seeing) and just to be safe I'm going to get the doctor now." This will save you from walking into a routine vaccine appointment with five minutes left on the clock, vaccines in hand, only to find your patient is suffering from a severe skin infection. This has happened to me more than once. It's very frustrating for everybody, including the pet owner.

10. **If you're administering an IV dose of an opioid, hold on tight!** I've only had it happen about a dozen times, but when it does, it can be disconcerting and even dangerous. A fraction of animals who receive IV injections of pain medications like morphine or hydromorphone will freak out. I would get upset every time it happened because I worried that, even though I was trying to alleviate pain, I was causing it instead. These animals appeared to be in agony. They would scream and fight with all their might to get away. Some of them tried to bite.

Then one fine day I got admitted to the ER myself

for severe, acute abdominal pain. I got an IV injection of hydromorphone. Lucky for me, unlike my patients, I understand English. The nurse warned me I would experience an intense sensation of squeezing and increasing heat moving up by body to my chest but that I shouldn't worry – it was just the hydro-morphone. If she hadn't told me this, I would have freaked out too. Even though being a patient in the ER is no fun, I was incredibly grateful to discover what it actually felt like to be injected with an opioid. Now I know it doesn't hurt – it just feels really weird and can be scary if you don't understand what's happening. Since you never know which one of your patients is going to go bananas when you give an IV opioid, make sure the person restraining understands how the pet might potentially react so they can hold on nice and tight.

11. **Steroids can make you (and your patients) crazy.** The disadvantage we have as veterinarians is our patients can't tell us how different drugs make them feel. (Which is why we don't learn these things in vet school. Well, at least I didn't!) Just like opioids, steroids can cause behavioral changes in pets - the effects just take longer to become observable. I had many clients come back to me after I'd prescribed steroids to their pets telling me they needed a different medication because the steroids were making their pet act weird. Sometimes they'd

complain their pet paced all night long. Of course, I would be willing to try another medication (though, depending on the condition, there often aren't good alternatives), but the truth is I didn't really believe the steroids were causing the behavioral changes the owners described.

And then, you guessed it, I got prescribed steroids for a severe allergic reaction and got to find out how they make you feel! Crazy. They make you feel crazy. And energized. No, not just energized. Energized in a crazy way. Manic. I felt like a slightly unhinged Superwoman for the first week. I had so much extra energy I accomplished three times more than any ordinary mortal could have accomplished within the same time period. The second week I just felt agitated and irritable and crabby. Now, in addition to forewarning pet owners that steroids can cause their pets to eat more and drink and urinate more, I also tell them that behavioral changes are possible as well. This doesn't mean steroids are bad and should never be prescribed. Every drug has side effects. But we prescribe them when the side effects are preferable to the condition we're trying to ameliorate. I was miserably itchy. I was tearing my skin off with my finger nails I was so itchy. The steroids stopped that. Given the choice to do it again, I would still take those steroids.

12. **Avoid diagnostic momentum.** Diagnostic momentum is a cognitive bias that assumes a

previous diagnosis is correct. Veterinarians frequently have to see patients seen by other veterinarians. We may be told by an owner what a previous veterinarian diagnosed, or we may have access to the patient's medical record and learn the diagnosis that way. Most of the time a previous diagnosis is correct, but medicine is an imperfect science practiced by imperfect beings on dynamic and complex living creatures. It's always possible that something else is going on.

Doctors who work in emergency or specialty medicine need to be especially aware of this potential bias since they frequently see patients transferred from other doctors. As a new grad you'll feel compelled to believe all the diagnoses made by other, more experienced doctors. It's also easier and faster to proceed along well worn paths, and inexperienced doctors are tempted more than most to do so because they typically feel they are already juggling more than they can handle. But this is one of the easiest medical errors to avoid, and the best way to avoid diagnostic momentum is to perform a thorough physical exam and get a full patient history from the owner as if you are the first veterinarian to have ever seen the patient. If you find anything inconsistent with the existing diagnosis, investigate further. It may just be your chance to feel like a hero.

13. **If you think you should use antibiotics, use them.** We've all heard the talk about increasing antibiotic resistance, and we all want to do our part not to contribute to that very real problem. However, as a new doctor, you may find yourself vacillating between giving an antibiotic because you think your patient might need one - and wanting to be a "good doctor" by not overprescribing antibiotics.

When I was a new ER vet, one of the relief vets working with me one day gave me a very long, passionate lecture about the evils of overprescribing antibiotics. Later that day, I performed a laceration repair on a dog that had been attacked by another dog. I placed a drain in the wound. I argued with myself for several minutes about whether I should put the dog on antibiotics or not.

On the one hand, I really thought I should prescribe antibiotics. On the other hand, what about what Dr. Jones told me? After all, I had thoroughly cleaned and debrided the wound. If I put him on antibiotics, is it possible that bacteria that were already resistant to the antibiotic might colonize the wound, resulting in a worse outcome? He was a young, healthy dog. Shouldn't his immune system be able to protect him? Fluid would be draining out of the wound through the drain I placed, therefore that fluid moving out of the dog should prevent bacteria from migrating into the dog, right? (For your reference, this is not true. Bacteria can migrate up the drain regardless of how much fluid is draining out.) The owners were going to have the drain removed by their day veterinarian in 3 days. He should be fine for that period of time. The day vet would reassess the wound again then.

I elected not to put the dog on antibiotics. Three days later my medical director called me into his office. The day vet had called upset that I hadn't put the dog on antibiotics. Thank goodness the dog was fine! I told my medical director why I had elected not to, and he was glad to hear I had at least thought about it and hadn't just forgotten, "But," he said, "you should have put that dog on antibiotics."

Of course I should have! I know that now! I'm positively horrified now that I sent that dog home without antibiotics. A lot of horrible things can happen to an open wound in three days, no matter how young and healthy a patient may be! But because I was new and wanted so much not to be a "bad doctor" contributing the problem of increasing antibiotic resistance, I talked myself out of using antibiotics when I should have! So, if you start having this conversation in your head - this "should I or shouldn't I prescribe antibiotics" conversation - just prescribe them.

14. **Buying time for the big, gaping "now what?"**
Whether it's the first time you're seeing a patient or you're performing a recheck exam, the next question is always "now what?" and the most notable person

waiting for the answer is the pet owner. The pet owner expects you to tell them what should be done next, and they expect you to tell them now. They don't understand that doctors derive their medical plans by weighing information from multiple sources (physical exam, client and patient history, test results) against a combination of their own medical knowledge and information looked up on-the-fly plus a risk-benefit analysis. This is serious mental acrobatics. For reasons discussed earlier, seasoned veterinarians can often perform this feat so quickly they have a medical plan in mind before the client even has a chance to ask "now what?," but the less experienced you are, the longer it will take to come up with a plan you feel comfortable with. Here are three ways to buy the time you need:

>*Diagnostic tests:* Blood work takes time, radiographs take time, cytology takes time. If the pet owner has authorized you to perform any diagnostic testing, even before the results are available you can use that time to look something up or to start thinking about your medical plan based on potential results. Furthermore, the time these tests take varies depending on the lab equipment, the number of support staff available, how busy the clinic is, and how complicated other cases in the clinic are. No one

can predict how long it will be before the test results are available. This brings me to the second way you can buy time.

Little white lies. Perhaps you have the radiographic, blood work and cytology results in hand but you're still not sure how you want to proceed. It may be a matter of simply needing to think about it a little longer, or you may need to look something up or ask another doctor who happens to be busy. There is no harm in poking your head into the exam room where your client is waiting to say, "I apologize for the wait, Mrs. Jones, but we're having some technical issues with some of our lab equipment so the blood work is taking longer than expected. Can I have someone bring you a cup of coffee or tea while you're waiting?" Other little white lies can include saying something lIke, "Mrs. Jones, before we decide what to do next I need to spend a little time in the doctors' office double checking something in Fluffy's history." Use your creativity and come up with a few of your own white lies that you can use to buy yourself a little extra time to think when needed.

Honesty. Honesty is a time buying tactic experienced vets feel comfortable with because they have the self-confidence to admit when they need more time to think. Depending on the situation and the rapport you feel with a pet owner, sometimes honesty is the best policy. There is nothing wrong with saying, "Mrs. Jones, I've never actually seen a case like this before so if you don't mind I'd like to ask Dr. Miller his opinion before proceeding." It's also perfectly reasonable for you to tell a pet owner that you'll need to do a little research before deciding what to do next. Most clients are perfectly happy to go home and wait for your follow up call. In fact, I find most of them appreciate knowing that a doctor is doing her best to be thorough, and that makes up for any delays or even the inconvenience of returning to the clinic to pick up medications later. Some doctors suggest owners leave their pet at the hospital to give the doctor more time, and again, most owners are fine with this.

15. **Do you feel lucky?** You're going to see other, more experienced doctors taking shortcuts or doing things in a way that you were taught not to. While there are many ways to do the same thing, and sometimes there are two or more correct ways to do something, just because you see other doctors doing something a certain way successfully, don't think you'll automatically enjoy the same success by imitating them. I've tried it, and here's what I learned: Some doctors are lucky. I'm not. Some doctors have the

Angel of Medicine sitting on their shoulders and they can get away with taking shortcuts and still get good outcomes. Perhaps it isn't magic. It may be due to a more experienced clinician having better intuition. Whatever the cause, before doing something the same way another doctor does it because it seems to work for them, ask yourself: Do you feel lucky?

16. **Place an IV catheter for every euthanasia, if possible, and give a sedative.** Euthanasia is a sacred duty. Someone is saying goodbye to someone they love. You want to do everything in your power to prevent this experience from being even more difficult for the owner than it already is. The hospital owner of the worst day practice ever used to give me a hard time for wanting to place IV catheters in patients that were going to be euthanized. It was a waste of time and money to him. He just injected directly into a vein.

Well, that may be fine if everything goes perfectly. But things going perfectly in medicine are the exception, not the rule. Having an IV catheter in place decreases the chances of causing the pet and the pet owner more distress. The pet owner is already distressed. Do you want to have to poke multiple times as you try to hit a vein on someone's beloved companion while they watch? What if the pet reacts to the needle stick and withdraws his leg? What if you only get half of the drug injected when the pet withdraws his leg?

This scenario is torture for a pet owner, and for the pet, and for the vet! Save yourself and everyone else the stress. Have an IV catheter placed in the pet in the treatment area, away from the owner. Test the IV catheter to ensure its patency (place your finger over the vein as saline is flushed through - you should be able to feel the saline moving through the vein - if you're able to push the saline but you don't feel it in the vein, the catheter is not properly placed and the saline may be leaking into the tissues under the skin). After the catheter is properly placed, carry the pet back to the room - either in your arms or on a stretcher. If the pet walks back to the room, the IV catheter may slip out of the vein.

If the owner asks why you want to place a catheter, tell them it's because you want to make sure this difficult experience isn't even more difficult for them or their pet, and having an IV catheter in place means you won't have to poke their beloved pet multiple times if he moves. If the owner asks why this has to be done in the treatment area instead of in front of them, just be honest: The technicians get very nervous if they have to place an IV catheter in front of an owner. When they're nervous, it's harder for them to correctly place the catheter, and that can make it more unpleasant for the pet.

Administer a sedative. When you become a veterinarian, you can ask other vets for their suggestions on which sedatives to use and how much. Some vets give the sedative before an IV catheter is placed. How much sedative you use will depend on whether the owner wants the pet to be awake or not when she's euthanized. A mild sedative will decrease the likelihood that the pet will struggle or vocalize during the euthanasia - both of which can be upsetting for an owner during an already very upsetting time.

Even with a sedative on board however, you should still prepare the pet owner for the possibility that their pet may drool, lick their lips excessively, struggle or vocalize when the drug is first injected. Let them know that you're injecting a barbiturate, and the drug can make animals feel "weird," (just like opioids can), but if their pet shows any of these behaviors it's because of this weird feeling and not because they're in pain. Also forewarn the pet owner that their pet may have tremors, or extend their limbs rigidly, may urinate or defecate, and may even show abnormal breathing after death - but that these are merely bodily reflexes. Tell them these things may not happen, but if they do, you want them to be prepared and you don't want them to be upset. There is no pain.

Another reason for placing an IV catheter is you can use a larger gauge needle to inject the euthanasia drug. (A larger gauge needle is even more difficult to use if you're just trying to inject directly into a vein, and your chances of "blowing the vein" increase.) The larger the gauge of the needle, the faster the drug can be delivered through the IV catheter, and the faster this drug is delivered, the less likely the pet will feel weird or vocalize.

Sometimes it's not possible to place an IV catheter. Sometimes an animal is so sick (or dehydrated) and their blood pressure is so poor that their veins are collapsed. You can't get an IV catheter in, and you can't just inject directly into the vein. Whenever a pet owner brings in a very sick animal for euthanasia, I always warn them that because of how sick their pet is, we may not be able to get venous access, and we may have to euthanize by injecting the euthanasia drug into the pet's abdomen. Warning pet owners of this possibility ahead of time will drastically reduce their distress if you do end up having to euthanize their pet in this way.

Of course, the exception is if a pet presents after suffering a severe trauma and is in terrible pain. In that case it's reasonable to try to inject the euthanasia drug into a vein - if you can - for the purpose of ending suffering immediately. Most euthanasia's do not present this way, however.

What Kind of Veterinarian Should You Be?

Who are you? What do you love? What do you hate? Do you get bored easily? Do you prefer variety in your day or would you rather have some predictability? Do you need a regular schedule in order to stay centered? Do you consider yourself a jack-of-all-trades, a renaissance man or woman, or would you rather be really good at one thing? How do you feel about chaos? How do you perform under pressure? Are you an introvert or an extrovert? How emotionally resilient are you? Do you like people? Are holidays a big deal to you or would you feel relieved to have an excuse not to partake? Are you a morning person or a night owl?

If you want to be a small animal veterinarian, the three

main categories for you to choose from are: Emergency medicine, general practice and specialty practice. Even though each focuses primarily on dogs and cats, there are significant differences between them. Which one you choose can strongly influence your sense of fulfillment and satisfaction in the future, depending on who you are and how you answer questions like the ones I just asked. Following is some top-line information on each of these three categories to help you consider which might best suit your personality.

Emergency Medicine

If you're a thrill seeking adrenaline junkie who thinks getting thrown into the deep end of a swimming pool sounds like fun, and you like variety and unpredictability, emergency medicine may be a great place for you to start your career - especially if you don't mind working overnights and holidays.

Experienced veterinarians are more likely to get the jobs they want – and most of them don't want to work graveyard shifts. If you're a fresh grad eager to begin earning a living and you're willing to endure a vampiric lifestyle, accepting a job as an overnight ER vet may be your fastest route to gainful employment. It's true that more ERs are looking for veterinarians who have done at least a one year internship, or who have other practice experience, however positions at ER hospitals are still available to the right new graduates when sufficient resources exist to offer mentorship and training. If you've got your heart set on starting out in ER without an internship, you may need to cast your net wider, and even consider moving out of state, but it can still be done. Several of my friends from vet school went into ER right after graduating just like I did.

Emergency medicine also tends to pay more. The average starting annual salary for new graduate small animal veterinarians in the United States, excluding those who pursue internship and residency training, has been holding steady since I graduated in 2011 at about $70,000. ER vets can start out at 80K to $100K a year, possibly more depending on the location. Rather than working four or five days a week as a typical day practice vet might, you'll be scheduled for ten to twelve 12-hour overnight shifts a month. Some ER vets like to work a lot of shifts in a row so they can have more days off in a row. Some prefer their work shifts and time off to alternate more frequently.

Starting your career in emergency medicine can make you a better doctor, too. ER hospitals tend to be better equipped, enabling a higher standard of medicine compared to day practices. As an ER vet you'll do many things you learned about in vet school - like ultrasound guided pericardiocentesis, inserting a long needle through the chest wall into the space surrounding the beating heart to draw out fluid. You'll place chest tubes. You'll perform c-sections and gastrotomies (surgical incision into the stomach, usually to remove a foreign body) and enterotomies (surgical incision into the small intestine). You'll diagnose and treat Addition's disease, diabetic ketoacidosis, hypoglycemia, toxicities, septic shock, head trauma, heart failure, immune mediated hemolytic anemia, pancreatitis, pyothorax, parvovirus, panleukopenia, and pneumonia. You'll learn how to communicate with pet owners about complex medical issues and you'll develop the ability to effectively direct a team of support staff under the most chaotic circumstances. If you stick with it long enough you'll eventually feel like you can handle anything that walks in the door – and that's an amazing feeling.

ER medicine provides excitement, variety and the intellectual stimulation of working with complicated and acute medical cases. Patients are triaged and the sickest are seen first. Doctors get to spend more time with them instead of being bound to a rigid schedule where every patient gets the same number of minutes regardless of presenting complaint. Unlike day practice vets, you don't have to have the same talk about vaccines and heartworm preventative twelve times a day, and you won't be managing chronic issues like allergies. Furthermore, if you're an introvert and don't really like small talk (like me), being an ER vet means forming close bonds and building long-term relationships with pet owners isn't a part of your job description. Your customers are other vets.

Your real clients are the general practice veterinarians in the area. It's their regular clientele you'll be seeing after those practices close for the night. Your medical records will be faxed to them, typically the morning after your shift. These records will tell the general practice veterinarians who you saw, what was wrong and what you did about it so they can follow up with their patients. Over time you'll learn about the preferences of the general practice vets in your area. For example, some will be able to do their own ultrasounds and will want you to refer patients needing that diagnostic test back to them. Others will be happy for you to refer those cases to a specialist.

Another advantage of ER medicine, especially if you work in a 24/7 hospital, is that another ER veterinarian will take over your hospitalized patients after your shift ends. As a new graduate, this gave me a lot of peace of mind. Knowing that diagnostic test results and treatment plans would be re-evaluated by a more experienced veterinarian after I went home made it a lot easier to sleep after my shifts. As just mentioned, outpatients I saw during the night would be followed up on by the day practice vets, so if I missed something, there was another chance for the pet to get the care he needed when the general practitioner read my record.

If all this sounds good to you, starting your veterinary career in emergency medicine could be a great choice. Even if you're an extrovert and would find forming bonds with pet owners easy, there's something to be said for not having to worry so much about that aspect of practice when you're just starting out. There are only two things that prevent me from unreservedly recommending emergency medicine to a new graduate. First, working nights is objectively bad for your health. It increases the risk of depression, obesity, diabetes, heart disease, and various types of cancer including breast cancer.[15] So you really need to be committed to managing and monitoring your health if you sign up for overnights.

According to my husband, I did it all wrong when I was an overnight ER vet. Instead of flipping my entire schedule upside down - that is, staying awake at night and sleeping during the day, even on my days off - I'd come home from an overnight, sleep four hours, then get up and try to act as if I hadn't been up all night. I'd go to bed around 10 or 11 o'clock and get up the next morning at 7 AM. I'd take a two hour nap in the afternoon, then head to work for another overnight. I thought this was an ideal way to live. Because I was sleeping less, I had more time!

But Alex tells me I was like a narcoleptic, constantly falling asleep, even in the middle of conversations. He also tells me my moods were erratic, and I can tell you, sticking to a healthy diet and exercise routine was almost impossible. It would have been better for my health had I flipped my entire schedule - so, if you take an overnight ER job - for your health and sanity, buy some blackout curtains, a white noise machine, and flip your entire schedule. Of course, you'll have to do your grocery shopping at a 24-hour Walmart and use the nearest urgent care facility as your GP, but... when your friends want to go out for a late dinner and then go dancing until the wee hours, you'll do great.

The second reason I hesitate to recommend starting out as an ER vet is because it will subject you to higher levels of emotional stress. You won't get the healthy puppy and kitten visits to brighten your shifts, like day practice vets do. Any puppies or kittens you see (unless you deliver them via an emergency c-section) are going to be sick, often very sick. A lot of your patients are going to be very sick. Being a slow turtle is hard enough as a day practice vet. But when you're an ER vet, and many of your patients are critically ill, being a slow turtle can make you feel like you're failing the animals you so much want to help.

I was astounded by the criticality and complexity of some of the cases I was responsible for. Patients presenting with dog bite wounds so extreme they needed vascular surgery (which I couldn't do), status epilepticus (prolonged and life threatening seizures) that could not be stopped with typical first or second line therapies, congestive heart failure with severe respiratory distress and pulse oximetry readings showing oxygenation levels in the 60's (a normal pulse oximetry range is 95% or above), dogs hit by cars with shattered pelvises, head trauma, diaphragmatic hernias... And all of these poor animals depending on me, a new graduate who had to look everything up, and whose entire surgical experience amounted to one enucleation in an otherwise stable patient with end stage glaucoma, a skin mass removal on my dermatology rotation, a c-section on a goat, a vasectomy on a bull, and a bunch of spays and neuters on young, healthy animals.

Most nights I had only one CVT (certified veterinary technician) working with me, and she was responsible for answering the door, checking in new patients, collecting payment for patients being discharged, answering the phone, and performing scheduled treatments on hospitalized patients - in addition to assisting me. One night we had a dog present in status epilepticus, and before I could get his seizure to stop - another dog in status epilepticus presented. As my technician was rushing the second seizuring dog back to the treatment area, a cat presented in such bad respiratory failure that his tongue was blue.

I had to stand between two adjacent treatment tables with one hand on each seizuring dog to prevent them from falling off the tables while my technician grabbed the cat, turned on the hospital's oxygen compressor, fed an oxygen line into the oxygen tent, and placed the suffocating cat inside. The phone was ringing throughout this ordeal, but obviously we just had to let it ring. Then a pregnant dog came in who needed an emergency c-section, which I performed - for the first time - after quickly reading about the procedure in my surgical textbook. (Some ERs have board certified veterinary surgeons on call, but mine didn't.)

At around three in the morning, it quieted down enough for me tackle a laceration repair on a dog who had been attacked by his housemate earlier that day. After the CVT helped me sedate and prep that dog, she went to catch up on treatments for other patients in the hospital when one of them started breathing abnormally and went into cardiac arrest. This little five foot nothing technician pulled a 120 pound Labrador out of his cage and began performing chest compressions.

I had to stop my suturing on the sedated patient, pull up an IV injection of epinephrine to push into the dying dog and then get a tube down his trachea so air could get into his lungs. After twenty minutes of CPR, without benefit of a defibrillator, I had to call the owners to break the news that their beloved dog had died. I did my best to comfort them while wondering if we could have saved him if we hadn't been so busy. The rest of my focus was on my sedated and half-sutured patient on the treatment table and whether he was going to wake up while I was on the phone.

It's difficult to describe how alone I felt being a new grad solely responsible for a hospital full of sick patients knowing that any kind of medical disaster could walk in the door at any moment. Even though my medical director gave me a generous six months of mentoring before I started working overnights by myself, it wasn't sufficient to prepare me for the weight of responsibility I had to shoulder. MDs who specialize in emergency medicine get *five years* of training before being left to their own devices in an ER, and even then, they are usually not the only doctor in the hospital. I do recommend that every veterinarian spend a couple of years practicing emergency medicine at some point in their careers, but unless you've got nerves of steel and very tough skin, you'll probably be better off beginning your career in general practice.

General Practice

I was delighted by how relaxed and friendly my clients were when I started general practice. Many people bringing sick pets to the ER are under emotional duress. They're scared, sad, angry, confused... But the majority of people I met as a day practice veterinarian were so cheerful and sunny it felt almost like each encounter came with a bouquet of daisies. It made me think maybe forming long-term relationships with clients wasn't so hard, even for an introvert like me. Sure, there were a few crab apples now and then, but no more than I'd expect to encounter as a coffee shop barista.

Another thing I loved about day practice was working with other veterinarians. I was accustomed to being the only doctor in the hospital and having to find answers to all my questions from books and the internet. Having other doctors to talk to as I worked my way through cases was a healing salve on the battle scars from my past life as a lone, midnight warrior. Lastly, a large proportion of pets I saw were perfectly healthy, and those pets who were sick generally had only mild to moderate signs of illness. That meant there was some wiggle room if the clients just wanted to try symptomatic or empirical treatment. Once in a while a critical case would come in, but this only happened once or twice a week.

These are all great reasons to start your career in

general practice, however, even though the average stress level will be lower than what ER vets experience, going straight from vet school to general practice may expose you to the highest levels of transition shock. If you did your clinical rotations as a fourth year veterinary student in a teaching hospital, what you're going to see in day practice could be about as far away from that as you can get while still remaining in the same country. Here is where it will be most important for you to remember to keep calm and make do with what you've got. You're going to have to learn a completely different way of practicing medicine than what you learned in vet school.

Some practices are well equipped, most are of moderate means, some operate with the bare bones minimum. Some practices are fully staffed with highly qualified and well trained certified veterinary technicians, some are under staffed and some will only have poorly trained, unqualified veterinary assistants to help you. (I know this because I was one of those poorly trained, unqualified veterinary assistants before I got into vet school.) Some practices are incredibly well managed with clear roles, responsibilities and workflow protocols. Others will operate without any apparent rhyme or reason and you'll battle all the chaotic forces of the universe until you gain enough of a foothold to impose your own order.

Every private veterinary hospital will be its own unique world. If you want to be good at making do with what you've got, wherever you end up, your first order of business should be familiarizing yourself with the resources you have on hand. Do an inventory of the equipment – from radiology to medical records to in-house lab equipment to syringes and types of IV fluids and fluid pumps available. Check the pharmacy for the kinds of medications you'll be able to send home with patients. Which local pharmacies are available for prescriptions you'll need to call in? Ask where other drugs like IV antibiotics, injectable steroids, diphenhydramine, lidocaine, and epinephrine are stored. Which controlled drugs are available? What policies and protocols are in place? What outside labs does the hospital use? Assess the skill level of the support staff. Who's great at patient restraint? Who's better at blood draws? Can they perform urinalyses? Cytology? Who assists with surgery? Observe the other doctors. Is one of them considered the go-to person for certain types of cases like orthopedic issues? Are there any nearby referral and emergency hospitals? What kind of specialists do they have on staff?

The second order of business is preparing yourself to see the types of cases you never learned about in veterinary school. Your vet school professors were either research oriented PhDs or they were board certified veterinary specialists. They taught you what they knew, but they probably weren't general practitioners. So you may remember the lecture on hip replacement surgery but what do you do for a kitten with a broken toe? You learned plenty about adenocarcinomas of the anal gland but what spectrum of size and shape fall into the category of normal anal sacs? And when you feel one, how do you know whether you should express it or leave it be? If you see a constipated cat without the infamous megacolon you heard so much about in vet school, what do you do? Maybe you'll try an enema. How much liquid should you use? What kind of liquid should you use? When will you know if it's worked?

Because the medicine you learn in veterinary school is so different from that of general practice, I'm inclined to say it's most important for a new grad to work with other doctors if they begin their careers as GPs. I've heard of new grads being hired by solo general practitioners and being left on their own from day one so their boss can take a badly needed vacation. This happened to one of my classmates. To me this seems akin to practicing for years for your first space flight as an astronaut only to find out on launch day you're going to have to pilot an airplane by yourself instead. Probably the best way to avoid having this happen to you is to make your expectations clear from the start: They won't leave you alone before you feel ready.

If you are working at a place where there are only one or two other doctors, it's conceivable that on some days you'll have to be the only doctor in the hospital. In this case, you'll want to be sure that another doctor is on-call to answer your questions by phone, and to come in to help if you get into trouble. The best case scenario if you start your career in general practice is to land your first job in a multi-doctor practice where you will never be the only doctor in the hospital.

Time management is also a completely different animal in general practice. In the ER, you see the sickest patients first and they get more of your time. In general practice, there's a set schedule and, depending on where you work, it's possible that all appointments may be given the same amount of time regardless of why the pet is being brought in. Although there seem to be more general practice walk-in clinics every year, most day practices are still appointment based. This can be a blessing, and it can be a curse.

A set schedule can be a blessing if you round with your team before appointments to develop your plans for controlling the controllable. A set schedule can be a curse because the uncontrollable happens every day. Walk-in emergencies, sick staff members, demanding clients, aggressive or uncooperative patients, previously stable in-hospital patients destabilizing, wellness visits turning out to be sick, sick visits turning out to be a lot sicker than expected... All of these unexpected issues must be addressed using minutes that have already been allocated to other appointments.

Time management in general practice requires an appreciation for the value of every minute. Just like people who appreciate the value of a dollar watch every dollar, a doctor who appreciates the value of a minute watches every minute. Minutes are the currency of your day. Spend them wisely and you might just end up with a few left over at the end of your shift. Spend them carelessly and you'll have to pay back the wasted minutes by staying late. Once in a while this can't be helped. But if you allow it to happen on a regular basis, you will burn out. You need to get out of the clinic on time so you can do things that help you recharge before having to come back to work the next day.

That being said, as a new grad, you should expect to stay late for the first few months. You'll have a steep learning curve to climb that includes not only learning how to practice medicine but also how to wisely use the resources at your disposal, how to manage your support staff, how to communicate with clients, and how to juggle your precious minutes in a dynamic environment. You won't be good at it in the beginning. As a new veterinarian, in order to do what must be done during hospital operating hours, like caring for patients, you'll have to put off writing medical records and making client callbacks until after the clinic has closed. But always remember that your goal is to eventually become so expert in managing your minutes that you accomplish what must be done during the day with enough minutes left over to complete your medical records and client callbacks before the hospital closes.

When you reach this level of time management expertise, staying after hours should happen very rarely. You'll know you've become a GP Time Management Expert when you stay on schedule, meet patient needs and client expectations, keep yourself and your support staff smiling, and make it home in time for dinner – all despite the uncontrollable. This requires discipline, diplomacy, the ability to creatively make do with what you've got, and practice... But once you get good at it, I promise, there's no better feeling in the world.

The last thing I want you to know about general practice is what I consider the most difficult aspect of being a GP. Nothing ever made me feel more liberated than when, as an ER vet, I got to say, "Please follow up with your regular veterinarian." Whether I was discharging a patient recovering from a serious illness like diabetic ketoacidosis or a patient with an ear infection, having no further medical responsibility for those patients' chronic medical conditions felt like joyfully running naked through a field of clover on a warm summer day.

Managing chronic medical conditions like diabetes and allergies is not necessarily intellectually difficult (although it can be). Mostly, it's emotionally difficult. Why? Because no matter how well you understand that these conditions can't be cured and must instead be managed, seeing the same patients for the same things over and over again can make you feel like a failure. Dogs with allergies get recurrent skin infections, even if they're on a good allergy management program. It can be extremely difficult to keep a cat's diabetes under control, even if you do everything right. We become doctors because we want to help and heal. Managing chronic conditions sometimes doesn't feel like we're doing either, even when we are. I think this is the toughest part of general practice.

Some key topics to pay extra attention to in veterinary school if general practice is your destination are parasitology, nutrition, reproduction and genetic disorders, geriatric medicine and physical therapy, behavior, dentistry, and vaccinology.[19] If you can do some additional reading on these topics while in school this could be very helpful to you when you begin general practice.

Another thing to think about as a future GP veterinarian is whether you might like to have a special focus. Do you want to be considered to "go-to" doctor in your practice for anything? Perhaps you'd like to be the best ultrasonographer in your practice, or the most skilled and knowledgeable about dentistry? Perhaps you'd like to get extra training so you can offer services like acupuncture or rehab therapy? Being to "go-to" doctor for something increases your value as an employee in the practice, while giving you the satisfaction that comes from further exploring specific medical interests.

Specialization

While emergency vets and general practitioners need to be (and hopefully enjoy being) jacks of all trades, if you'd prefer to narrow your focus and get really good at a shorter list of skills, specialization could be right for you. You'll naturally want to choose a specialty based on your interests. Go to the AVMA website and search for "veterinary specialists" for a list of recognized specialists and a brief description of their roles.

You should also take into consideration how much

variety you crave. Some specialties get more variety than others. Internists, criticalists and pathologists probably get the most. Orthopedic surgeons and dermatologists probably get the least. Your need for variety is an important consideration and I think many doctors, including MDs and DOs, realize too late that their chosen specialty, while theoretically interesting, in reality requires them to see a small handful of similar cases over and over again.

For example, an MD might choose to specialize in endocrinology because she thinks it's fascinating. Endocrinology is fascinating! Theoretically. It's all about feedback loops between different glands and organs in the body. But in practice, most of an endocrinologist's patients are diabetics. Alex considered specializing in neurology because the subject is vast and interesting. He's happy he became an internist instead though because it turns out the neurologists he knows spend most of their time diagnosing strokes.

A veterinary orthopedic surgeon spends most of her time doing knee and hip surgeries. A veterinary dermatologist spends most of his time seeing allergy cases. Although they specialize in a field that encompasses a variety of pathologies, common things are common - and they see them commonly. So it's important for you to know that some specialties will offer more variety, while some will offer the opportunity to become masterful at a narrower skill set. You just need to know which fits your personality better.

Specialists are also more likely to "figure it out and fix

the patient." A specialist's additional education and training enables him to more effectively pursue advanced diagnostics. This isn't to say every client seeing a specialist will follow the specialist's recommendation. In fact, according to a recent survey published in the *Journal of the American Veterinary Medical Association*, a greater proportion of specialist responders than general practitioner responders indicated "client financial limitations adversely affected their ability to provide patient care."[2]

This isn't surprising if you consider that costs of specialist care are inherently higher than costs of care provided by general practitioners, so naturally a greater proportion of clients seeing a specialist will be limited by those higher costs. Yet when a client is able and willing, the path to a definitive diagnosis on a complex medical case frequently leads to a specialist.

About a third of veterinary students are now pursuing advanced study like specialty board certification.[1] In private veterinary practice, surgeons and internists are the most common specialists. Board certified veterinary specialists *can* attain incomes two or even three times higher than that of general practice associates, and *can* make as much as practice owners but without the financial investment and risk that accompanies practice ownership.[6]

For this fact alone, I'd like to be able to say that everyone wanting to become a small animal veterinarian should pursue specialization. Unfortunately, reality won't support this recommendation. The Veterinary Internship and Matching Program listed 906 internship positions but only 263 residency positions in 2011.[4] There aren't enough residency positions to accommodate everyone who completes an internship, much less every graduating veterinarian. Clearly, not everyone wanting to become a small animal veterinarian can pursue specialization. The advice I gave in Book 2 about trying to be less of a perfectionist and not focusing so heavily on test grades may not apply if specialization is your goal. It's even more competitive than getting into vet school.

It's also important to consider that some veterinary specialties, such as surgery and internal medicine, are currently in demand and pay better. If you specialize in these fields, and present market circumstances hold steady, you're likely to find a good paying position in a private hospital. Specialists in private practice however are going to feel the hit of an economic recession earlier and more severely than their counterparts in general practice.[5] Other veterinary specialties, like anesthesiology, are typically needed only in teaching hospitals (board certification is one route to working in academia). Competition for those jobs will be stiff, salaries will be far less than that of a veterinary surgeon, and you may have no other choice but to go where you're offered a job.

My sister in-law has a PhD in Medieval History from Oxford University. She is published. She is brilliant. However, as you can imagine, good jobs for experts on Medieval History are few and far between. She was extremely fortunate to be offered a tenured position in an obscure town in Texas where the closest city of interest, San Antonio, is two hours way. If you choose to specialize in something with low market demand because you love it, you need to be willing to work hard enough to make yourself competitive, and prepare to choose between doing what you love and living where you want.

If you already know you want to specialize, as soon as you start veterinary school, seek out specialists in your area of interest and start a dialogue. Let them know you want to be what they are. Ask for their advice and help. Maintain a relationship with them as you progress through vet school. Their guidance can greatly enhance your chances of getting one of those rare, coveted residency positions.

It's Never Too Late to Change Your Mind

Many small animal veterinarians switch between general practice and emergency medicine during their careers. There are even veterinarians who went directly into private practice after graduating and then, after a few years, decided to pursue specialization and were able to land a residency position. This isn't the traditional path to specialization but it is possible. So remember, no matter where you begin, you can always change your mind.

Additional Options to Consider When You're More Experienced

Following are six additional categories to consider as a small animal veterinarian. These categories are either not possible (ABVP specialization) or are not recommended (relief work, shelter medicine, hospice, practice ownership, mobile practice) for new graduates, but they are options you may want to consider after you have attained sufficient experience.

Relief veterinarian

Relief veterinarians are independent contractors. They fill in when other veterinarians go on vacation or take time off for other reasons. Most relief veterinarians charge an hourly rate. These rates vary depending on where they practice, and also may vary depending on the type of shift they've agreed to do. For example, some relief veterinarians charge more to fill in on ER shifts than for a shift at a day practice. They may also elect to charge more for taking a shift on late notice.

One advantage of being a relief veterinarian is that you are your own boss. You decide when and where you will work, for how much and for how long. Another two advantages of doing only relief work is that you won't have to concern yourself with intra-hospital politics and you won't be responsible for the ongoing management of chronic medical conditions. The disadvantages are that you must pay for your own licensing fees, association dues, continuing education, and health insurance, you must do your own marketing, and you theoretically have less security than a veterinarian working on salary at one animal hospital. Nonetheless, there are many experienced small animal veterinarians who have chosen to do only relief work. Some of them pick up relief shifts in just one area, for example, the southwest suburbs of Chicago. Other relief veterinarians are licensed in multiple states and serve a larger geographical area.

The reason relief work is something you should consider only after you have several years of experience is that relief veterinarians need to perform as effective practitioners in a multitude of different environments. They must feel comfortable practicing despite their unfamiliarity with hospital staff, protocols, equipment, medical records systems, etcetera. This is too much to expect of a new graduate who is just learning how to apply his academic knowledge to real world situations.

Shelter Medicine

Shelter medicine is quite a different animal from traditional small animal practice. Yes, you are still treating individual animals, but you are also responsible for decisions that affect the health and wellbeing of every animal that comes to your shelter. This is called population medicine, and it covers broad topics such as how to prevent and handle infectious disease outbreaks. Most shelter veterinarians also need to feel comfortable doing large numbers of spay and neuter surgeries every day. Some shelter veterinarians report doing up to 60 surgeries per day! This requires extensive surgical experience and confidence, something new graduates will naturally lack.

One important aspect to consider if you think shelter medicine might be a career option for you in the future is that many shelter veterinarians have to perform euthanasia on homeless animals. Sometimes, euthanasia will be performed because an animal is injured, severely ill and suffering. Sometimes euthanasia will be performed because an animal is considered aggressive and dangerous. But sometimes euthanasia may have to be performed on healthy animals simply because there is not enough space in the shelter for everyone and there are not enough people looking to adopt a shelter animal.

There are no-kill shelters, of course, but the reality remains that while healthy animals may not be euthanized at a no-kill shelter, when a no-kill shelter is at capacity, there must be somewhere else for homeless animals to be taken, and often that is a municipal shelter that has no choice but to euthanize healthy animals when they run out of space. If you want to become a veterinarian because you want to help animals, being a shelter vet may enable you to do a great deal of good, but in order to make a positive difference in the wider world, you must be able to emotionally withstand the suffering and sadness of every individual homeless animal, some of whom you will not be able to help. You'll also have to be involved in cases of animal abuse and neglect. You may be able to make a positive difference, but you'll also be exposed to some very distressing situations.

Shelter medicine is not something I learned anything about in veterinary school. In the years since I graduated however, more shelters are employing veterinarians and therefore some veterinary schools may offer lectures on shelter medicine. The University of Florida offers online courses in shelter medicine that can lead to a Master's Degree or a Graduate Certificate. Theoretically, these can be earned concurrently as you pursue your DVM, but please speak with the administrators of your school if this is something you want to pursue. You will need their support to balance the rigors of veterinary school with additional online courses. Some veterinary schools have even started offering residencies in shelter medicine, including the University of Florida, Tufts Cummings School of Veterinary Medicine and UC Davis.

ABVP specialization

The American Board of Veterinary Practitioners has options for small animal veterinarians who wish to become board certified in Canine and Feline Practice, Feline Practice or Shelter Medicine. Interested veterinarians must have six years of related, full-time experience to qualify for these programs. This type of board certification doesn't lead to significantly higher wages such as would be expected if you were to become a board certified surgeon, but for those interested in higher learning pertaining specifically to these areas of interest, this is the route to consider. For more information visit the ABVP website.

Practice Ownership

Besides becoming a board certified veterinary surgeon or internist, probably the next best chance for making enough money to earn financial freedom is owning your own practice. According to a recent online survey, over 80% of veterinary students who responded indicated they wanted to own their own practice someday, while only 50% of responding practicing veterinarians reported wanting their own practice someday.[17]

As a veterinary student, I too dreamed of owning my own practice but have since changed my mind. I speculate that many vet students have a change of heart on this topic once they start practicing because they quickly realize that just being an associate veterinarian working for someone else taxes their ability to maintain a good work-life balance. Another reason associate veterinarians eschew practice ownership is that, as with any business venture, while it may lead to financial freedom, it also has the potential to lead to financial ruin. If you're already carrying a hundred thousand dollars in student loan debt (or more), it's hard to take the plunge into several more hundreds of thousands of dollars of business loan debt.

However, if you've got courage, vision and the willingness to work very hard for a very long time, practice ownership offers the chance to create something just the way you want it, to practice medicine your way, to make the rules, to hire who you want (and fire who you want) and maybe even to make a good living while you're at it. Just set your expectations appropriately. It can take many years before all your hard work pays off. Here are three basic choices for owning your own practice.

> **Buy-in:** Your employer may offer the option of buying an ownership share in her practice. This can be the fastest, easiest path to owning your own little piece of the pie. You may be able to negotiate a payment plan that involves a percentage of your check going toward the buy-in over a specified period of time. Once you buy in, a percentage of the profits of the practice belong to you in proportion to your ownership share. If it's a profitable practice, this can make a big difference in your earnings.
>
> While I recommend focusing on building your medical knowledge and skills for several years before adding the additional demands that will come with owning your own practice, there is even more reason to wait before buying into someone else's practice. Entering into a business partnership is like getting married, except if things don't work out, it's often easier to get out of a marriage than a business partnership. You need an extended period of time to adequately

assess whether the practice owner would be a compatible business partner based on her personality, her work ethic and sense of fairness, her standards of medicine and practice management philosophy - and judging these accurately requires experience as a practicing veterinarian.

If after sufficient consideration you decide to proceed, there are three major elements that should be addressed in the practice ownership agreement.[8] First, how will compensation be calculated? In addition to the obvious, the agreement should include specifics on how each owner will be compensated for time and work done related to managing the practice. I've heard horror stories from vets whose business partners let them do the lion's share of the work without additional compensation or even acknowledgement. Second, what exactly are the management responsibilities of each owner? Who makes which decisions as to how the practice should be managed? Which decisions require consensus and which don't? Third, what's the exit strategy? What happens if one partner wants out? Or if a partner dies? Even if it looks to you that the agreement is fair and covers what needs to be covered, do not sign an ownership agreement without legal counsel.

Buy-out: Buying an existing practice can be the least risky road to practice ownership. As you go through the due diligence process you'll find out how profitable the practice is and, perhaps more importantly, how the practice has performed over many years. This is information that will help you calculate whether you can make the monthly payments on the business loan and support yourself (including making your student loan payments). Buying an existing practice also usually means you're getting a turn-key operation, meaning all the equipment, computers and software, employees, and systems and protocols are already in place.

The disadvantage of buying an existing practice is, if there's anything you want to change, you'll have to go to bat against the legacy infrastructure. "Legacy infrastructure" is a term most often used to describe existing computer systems that a company depends upon but that also impede improvements, such as servers that are incompatible with the latest, greatest business software applications.

I like to apply the term more broadly. In the truest sense of the term, let's say the existing computer system of the practice is outdated and in need of replacement, but it's what's keeping the hospital running. For a non-computer related analogy, what if you want to add more exam rooms but can't afford to shut down the hospital while construction is performed? What if you want to make policy changes but the employees who came with the hospital don't like your ideas? What if you want to raise prices but the clients protest? These are all "legacy infrastructure" challenges. You can however, negotiate with the owner of the practice to partner with you in implementing some changes, such as policy changes or price changes. Employees and clients may be less resistant to these changes if they are advocated by the original owner, with whom they have a trusted relationship.

There are companies that specialize in helping veterinarians purchase a practice. Many can evaluate the practice, provide legal representation, and even help you obtain a business loan. Just Google "buying a veterinary practice" and you'll get enough search results to start you in the right direction. Just remember to do your homework on any company you're considering, as well as the process in general. The Veterinary Information Network (VIN) can be a great resource where you can ask fellow veterinarians for advice and recommendations on this topic.

Build from scratch: If you've got an entrepreneurial spirit and you dream of owning your own practice isn't merely about financial freedom but also encompasses less quantifiable rewards such as creative expression and the fulfillment that comes from building something yourself, this is likely the option for you. It's the most costly and most risky of all the options, but I know veterinarians – including those who have graduated within the past ten years - who have gone this route and succeeded.

Building your own practice from scratch is such a massive project, with so many different pieces and parts, the best advice I can give you on this subject is to urge you to watch the online video series by veterinary architect Mark Hafen. The series is broken into six chapters and covers topics from planning and zoning issues to choosing a contractor to what a bank will want before qualifying you for a loan. Watching the series won't give you a PhD in building a veterinary practice, but it will give you a realistic idea of the scope of the endeavor. It is not for the faint of heart. Google, "Mark Hafen's Complete Guide to Building Your Veterinary Hospital" or use the direct link at http://www.realize.vet/book3-resources

There are two additional ownership options I'd like to mention. They are less likely to generate the significant wealth associated with the concept of financial freedom but they're also less risky financially, and they have a greater potential for allowing you to sustain a healthy work-life balance, despite being a business owner. As with the other ownership options I've discussed, several years of medical experience are recommended before going it alone in either of these two practice ownership models.

> **Mobile General Practice:** As a mobile general practitioner, you can operate anywhere on the spectrum between practicing out of a decked out, converted RV with its own surgical suite (these are available for sale from multiple manufacturers including a company in my home state of Arizona called Magnum Mobile) to practicing out of the back of the old Honda Civic hatchback you inherited from your grandmother. Perhaps you want to offer on-call emergency door-to-door service with the option of performing an emergency c-section on site if that's what's needed? Or maybe you just want to do wellness exams and vaccines? Or maybe you'll do wellness exams but also offer emergency pet taxi services to your patients when they need to go to the ER? It's all completely up to you. Be as creative as you like.
>
> Many mobile practitioners enjoy being able to see patients in their own homes, and the patients often like it better too. It also gives the veterinarian an opportunity to develop more meaningful relationships with their clients, and

being able to provide medical care to pets whose owners can't easily bring them to a hospital, like the physically handicapped or elderly, can be emotionally rewarding too. Just take into consideration the demographics of where you plan to do this.

In more rural areas you'll have to drive longer distances between appointments, limiting the number of patients you can see in a day, increasing the cost of travel and decreasing your income. In a busy city, heavy traffic could cause similar challenges. I would wager the best place to be a mobile GP is a nice, middle class suburb. Also, the fewer services you offer, the more important it will be for you to work with local brick and mortar practices to ensure your patients have access to full spectrum medical care.

Mobile Hospice Veterinarian: I spoke earlier about my experiences with hospice when my father was dying. Although I wish he could have been spared the five days of suffering as he waited for death, it was a welcome alternative to prolonging a life devoid of agency and happiness. However, I do believe there are circumstances when hospice is preferable to euthanasia, especially in veterinary medicine. I know this may sound like a contradiction of sentiments previously expressed, but bear with me.

A great proportion of my father's suffering during his last days was emotional and psychological. It was due to his capacity to understand he would never walk again, never move again, never speak again. He understood his life was over, that all the wonderful dreams he had about his future in Flagstaff, about growing papaya trees, about sitting on his sun drenched patio as he lovingly watered his herb garden, would never come to pass. He understood he was waiting for death.

Animals like dogs and cats don't suffer in this way. While they do have the capacity to suffer emotionally and psychologically, this kind of suffering occurs when they can't be where they feel most safe and comfortable, when they can't be with the people they love. If a dog or cat were to be admitted for in-hospital hospice, as my father had been, I'd have considered it cruel. But veterinary hospice is a service provided in the animal's home environment. (While residential hospice programs do exist for animals, I am not an advocate for the prolonged stress I believe this would cause a pet. Furthermore, there have been cases where residential hospice programs have been used as fronts for animal hoarders who claim to be against euthanasia, using it as an "excuse for the poor condition of the hoarded animals."[13])

If an animal diagnosed with a terminal illness can be kept physically comfortable at home, this is a reasonable alternative to euthanasia. If the animal is later determined to be suffering despite all efforts made to mitigate her pain, euthanasia remains an option.

While the concept of human hospice dates back to the 1960s, veterinary hospice is relatively new. It wasn't discussed while I was in veterinary school and I am only now learning about it. Up to this point I'd considered euthanasia the only option for a terminal diagnosis. Sometimes, if the pet wasn't in unmanageable pain, I would offer clients the choice of waiting a day or two to give them a little more time with their pet at home. Usually this was so other family members and friends could say goodbye. But, having little knowledge about, or experience with, veterinary hospice, I never offered it as an alternative to euthanasia, and retrospectively I can think of multiple cases where it could have been a better alternative.

In an older dog, acute bleeding into the abdomen in the absence of trauma or exposure to rat poison is most likely due to an aggressive cancer called hemangiocarcinoma. The malignant cells arise from blood vessel walls, and as the tumor grows, eventually a fatal bleed occurs. When the love of my life, my dog, Monte, developed hemoabdomen at the age of fourteen, I knew it was a death sentence. I was scheduled to work at the ER that night, and though I begged my medical director to find someone else to take my shift, he was unable to. Alex drove me to work while I held Monte on my lap. I euthanized the best friend I've ever had in my life before my 12-hour overnight shift. Even though I was able to hold Monte in my arms, to thank him for loving me, to thank him for being my best friend before I pushed an overdose of barbiturate into his vein and felt his body go limp in my arms, knowing what I know now, I would have chosen hospice instead.

Hemangiosarcoma can cause multiple, non-fatal bleeds over time before the final fatal bleed occurs. While the tumors themselves can be painful, bleeding to death is not. You simply become progressively tired and weak until you lose consciousness. I could have spared Monte the stress of being driven to the hospital and dying in an unfamiliar place. Instead, I could have given him the gift of days or even a week of my undivided attention and love at home, in his favorite bed, surrounded by his toys, with all the pain medication necessary to keep him comfortable and calm. I chose to go to work that night because I thought euthanasia was the only option, but had I been better informed, I wouldn't have asked my medical director to try to find someone to take my shift. I would have told him he had to.

I'm telling you this story not only to demonstrate how veterinary hospice can be better than euthanasia for some terminally ill pets, but also to help you understand how much better it can be for owners as well. Making the decision to euthanize a beloved pet can cause feelings of intense guilt, especially when the euthanasia is performed when the pet is alert and showing no signs of severe discomfort. Additionally, having a pet euthanized in the hospital increases the stress for the owner as well as the pet. Yes, there are times when euthanasia is the best option, but now you know it isn't the only option.

Veterinary hospice requires a very strict set of circumstances. The hospice veterinarian needs to make frequent visits to the home to check on the patient in case adjustments in medication are needed, and must be available 24/7 should an emergency situation arise. Owners must be able and willing to provide all the needed supportive care at home. Owners who cannot take time off from work, or elderly owners unable to perform the physical tasks necessary to support the pet at home, may preclude hospice as an option.

When you begin practicing, find out if there are any hospice veterinarians practicing in your area. I recommend meeting with them if possible to learn about their services so you can feel comfortable recommending them when you encounter a pet and a family you think would benefit from veterinary hospice. You can also learn more about veterinary hospice from them with an eye on considering it as a potential career alternative in the future. I don't recommend it for inexperienced veterinarians however because it requires exceptional medical judgment and intuition, as well as the kind of client communication skills that take years to build.

Several years ago, veterinarians Dr. Dany McVety and Dr. Mary Gardner partnered to create a veterinary hospice franchise called Lap of Love. Currently there are veterinarian Lap of Love franchise owners providing veterinary hospice care in twenty-nine states across the country. The franchise offers education, training and other forms of support to its franchise owners. Lap of Love even offers a 1-week externship opportunity to veterinary students. This might be a great thing to do during your summer vacations between first and second or second and third year of vet school (there's no summer vacation after third year). Google Lap of Love veterinary hospice externship or follow the link provided on my website at www.realize.vet/book3-resources You don't have to be a Lap of Love franchise owner in order to offer veterinary hospice care, but it's one available option that could ease your transition into an emerging field within veterinary medicine.

Beyond Small Animal Medicine

Small animal veterinary medicine is a relatively narrow focus within the wider field of veterinary medicine. It's just one option among many that exist for those earning a DVM degree. Other kinds of veterinarians do very different things. They lead very different lives. They took very different roads to get where they are. There are horse vets, farm vets, zoo vets, wildlife vets, vets who specialize in exotic species, vets who work at Sea World, vets who work in industry, pharmaceuticals, government, the army, and in non-profit. There are vets who do research or teach. If you'd like to hear more about veterinarians doing all sorts of different work, go to my website and check out my podcast.

How to Decide Where (and Where NOT) to Practice

The hospital where you choose to begin your career can have a big impact on the trajectory your career takes. A bad experience right out of school can cause serious emotional trauma.[5] If you listen to my podcast, you'll hear a recurring theme from the doctors I've interviewed. Many of them had very negative experiences with their first employers. Some veterinarians have even chosen to leave the profession altogether because their initial experiences as new veterinarians were so negative. I know that as a new graduate you're probably going to feel lucky if anyone wants to hire you at all. That's how I felt. I know you may feel financial pressure to begin working as soon as possible. I did. But it will never be more important for you to work in a positive and supportive environment than in your first several years out of school. All the self-care in the world won't do you any good if the environment you work in is toxic.

In a paper entitled, *"Beyond Kale and Pedicures: Can We Beat Compassion Fatigue?"* the author points out that, all too often, people who work in the helping professions are not suffering from insufficient yoga. They are suffering because the culture of the places where they work are toxic, the workloads are unreasonable, they aren't given the training and support they need, making it impossible for them to provide good quality care. They work at hospitals where they are chastised for insufficiently increasing revenues, while being forced to wear buttons that proclaim "we provide compassionate care."

The self-care practices I recommend in Book 1 of this series are meant to help you cope with the emotional difficulties that come with being a veterinary doctor - sick patients, suffering, sadness, your own imperfections, the imperfections of medicine, transition shock... These are the unavoidable downsides of being a doctor - any kind of medical doctor. These practices could have helped me immensely when I first started my career as a veterinarian - because the hospital where I worked was a good hospital.

But the practices in Book 1 are not going to be sufficient to protect you from burnout and depression if you don't avoid the downsides of this career that *can* be avoided. You can avoid working in toxic environments. You can avoid working for a boss that sees you only a revenue generating machine instead of a human being.

You can avoid working at hospitals that prioritize making money over practicing good medicine. You can avoid working at hospitals that make it impossible to practice good medicine, or compassionate medicine. You can avoid working at hospitals that make it impossible for you to have a healthy work-life balance.

Even if you need to live in your parents' basement for a while, I strongly advise you to be very selective about where you begin your career as a veterinarian. If you don't want to stay with your parents, rent a cheap apartment with three of your vet school classmates and wait tables or be a coffee barista until you find a good hospital. There is a six month grace period after you graduate vet school before you have to start making payments on your student loans. Don't rush.

If you feel that you have to accept a position at a hospital that is not ideal, do not resign yourself to staying there. Make sure you have a game plan for moving on to something better at the earliest opportunity. Consult a lawyer before signing any contract to ensure you don't end up legally trapped in a place that makes you unhappy. I know vets this has happened to.

All this being said, gauging whether or not a practice is a good place to work can be challenging even for experienced veterinarians. It's virtually impossible for a brand new graduate to accurately assess a potential employer without the insight of experience. So, until you develop your own, I will give you mine, as well as what I've gathered from other experienced vets, mostly in the form of important questions you should ask potential employers. You'll have to weigh the information provided in the following sections against your own situation. For example, if you're starting out in an urban or highly populated suburban area, more choices will be available to you than if you live in a rural area. Taking into consideration your own circumstances, use the information in these sections in conjunction with your own judgment as you look for your first job.

First Impressions

In the U.S. or Canada, the red and white AAHA (American Association of Animal Hospitals) accreditation sticker in the window is a positive sign. Unlike human hospitals, animal hospitals are not required to be accredited and only 12-15% of animal hospitals in the U.S. and Canada are AAHA accredited. AAHA accredited hospitals adhere to the highest standards of veterinary care and are evaluated on over 900 different standards.

A good hospital will look and smell clean, both in the lobby, and in the areas of the hospital the public doesn't get to see. The receptionist should act welcoming and greet you professionally. Unless you're standing in the back of a line, the receptionist should acknowledge your presence even if he or she is busy, and you'll hear something to the tune of, "I'm sorry for the wait. I'll be with you shortly." You should not be made to wait more than fifteen minutes without apology or explanation (unless a critical emergency has presented). Other doctors and support staff working there should appear happy, even if busy (unless a euthanasia has just been performed or a critical emergency has presented). A mutual respect should be evident between all staff members. People you pass in the hallways should make eye contact and smile.

Unless your interviewer is a doctor, you should be addressed as "Doctor." If your interviewer is a doctor, and still addresses you as "Doctor," even better. (If you want to be perceived as respectful and considerate, you should always address doctors as "Doctor" unless or until invited to do otherwise, even after you become a doctor.) Your interviewer should appear friendly and seem genuinely interested in you. Your interviewer should not appear hurried or distracted. Your meeting should not be repeatedly interrupted. Deviation from this description doesn't necessarily mean the hospital isn't a good one, but it should increase your scrutiny as it may indicate potential underlying mismanagement. If the place looks and smells like a chaotic, unhappy zoo – it probably is – and it's unlikely to change, no matter what they tell you.

Questions to Ask

Following are a list of suggested questions to ask during an interview, along with an explanation of why I think they're important. A lot of these questions may seem hard-hitting. Asking them requires some courage. But a good hospital will be pleased to answer these questions and will consider them a sign that you're a conscientious doctor looking for long-term employment at a place where you can practice high quality medicine. Employers will ask questions to determine whether you're a good fit for their hospital. You have the right to ask questions to ensure they're a good fit for you as well. You may not be able to ask all of these questions, but at least choose the ones that are priorities for you and ask them first.

1. *I know that as a new graduate I'm going to need mentoring. Why is your hospital interested in hiring a new graduate despite the extra effort that will be involved?* With this question you're looking for your interviewer's reaction. Did it catch them off guard? If so, that could indicate they're just looking for any doctor, and they may have no formal plans for mentoring a new grad. What you'd like to hear as a response to this question is that they believe it's part of their professional responsibility to mentor new grads when they can, and they are looking for someone who wants to grow with their organization.

2. *I'm committed to becoming the best veterinarian I can. I know that an important part of achieving that objective is going to be my willingness to take a proactive role as a mentee. What protocols does your hospital have in place for mentorship and how can I contribute to help ensure the most successful outcomes?* Ideally, the hospital will have a written

plan for mentorship that will include roles and responsibilities of the mentor and mentee, expectations, goals, milestones, and a set schedule for ongoing evaluation of progress. Many hospitals, even good ones, will not. What you're trying to determine with this question is whether they would be open to collaborating with you to develop a formal, written mentorship plan based on your own professional goals. Check the AAHA website for more information on mentoring guidelines or find the direct link at www.realize.vet/book3-resources

3. ***Do you have an orientation plan for new doctors?*** You'll need some time to familiarize yourself with the hospital before you can start seeing appointments. Ideally, they have an employee handbook that discusses hospital culture, administrative procedures, roles, responsibilities, and expectations, but you'll also need someone to show you around. Remember what I said about learning to make do with what you've got? They should have some plan for showing you what they've got, where it is and how to use it.

4. ***What are your expectations in terms of how long it should take me to become fully autonomous? For example, if I were to hypothetically start working here today, what might be the earliest date at which I might find myself to be the only doctor in the hospital?*** This is to reduce the chances you'll be left to fend for yourself before you're ready. Unless it's a

big enough hospital where there's never only one doctor there (which is the best case scenario), you want them to say it depends on when you feel you're ready. At minimum they should have someone available to take your questions by phone until you're ready to practice without a net, and you should never be expected to perform surgeries without on-site assistance from another doctor until you feel comfortable doing those surgeries on your own.

5. **Why are you hiring a new doctor?** Are they expanding or are they replacing someone who's left? Why did that doctor leave? This is another question where you're really looking at how the interviewer reacts. If the interviewer behaves as if they're trying to hide something, they may be trying to replace someone who left for reasons associated with how the hospital is managed. Potential employers will probably want a list of references from you. How about asking them for references too - from doctors who used to work there.

6. **How long have the other doctors been with this hospital?** It's a good sign if the other doctors have been with this hospital for several years. If the interviewer is reluctant to answer this question or you learn that other doctors have been there for less than a year, this may be cause for concern.

7. ***Will I have the opportunity to speak with any of the other doctors?*** Obviously, the only right answer to this question is "yes," so again, the point here is to see how the interviewer reacts. You're looking for an attitude of openness.

8. ***How long have the support staff been with this hospital?*** See the explanation for question #6.

9. ***What is the support staff to doctor ratio?*** 2:1 or greater is what you want to hear. Two support staff <u>solely</u> devoted to helping you, plus another person acting as a "floater" (a floater chips in wherever they are needed throughout the day) is excellent. 1:1 plus a floater may be acceptable depending on how busy the practice is, how skilled the support staff are, and how well the practice is run.

10. ***How many of the technicians are certified or licensed?*** The more the better, but certainly the number will depend on the size of the practice. If the answer is "zero," unless this is a practice in a rural area or an area where, for whatever reason, licensed veterinary technicians are hard to come by, I'd be concerned about how highly this hospital values quality of care.

11. ***What is the general skill level of the support staff?*** Can they do blood draws, place IV catheters, run blood work, take radiographs, program IV fluid

pumps, read fecals and urinalyses, or do the doctors typically perform those tasks? If you have to do these things as a doctor, your ability to practice good medicine will be diminished, and the busier the practice, the more diminished your ability to practice good medicine will be. A poorly trained support staff may also indicate insufficient dedication to employee growth and satisfaction.

12. **What training protocols do you have in place for the support staff?** Good hospitals will have clear and written expectations of specific skills for different support staff positions, and they will have a system in place for teaching and evaluating those skills.

13. **What improvements is this hospital currently trying to implement and how are you going about it?** No matter how good the hospital, there will always be room for improvement, and the best hospitals are always trying to improve. Whether they're hoping to make their inventory management more efficient or they're experimenting with tactics to improve employee morale or they're in the process of creating a set of client education handouts for common pet health issues or they're working toward AAHA certification, you want to hear evidence they're not stagnant and smugly satisfied with the status quo.

An explanation of *how* they are trying to implement changes will give you a peek into their management philosophy. Ideally the answer will reflect a desire for employee engagement and openness to employee contribution. You may want to ask directly how they handle employee suggestions for improvement because you want to work at a hospital that empowers its employees to make positive changes. You will want to continually improve yourself as a veterinary doctor. This is very hard to do if you work at a hospital that isn't dedicated to its own continual improvement.

14. ***How does your hospital handle inter-personal conflict?*** You want to know that some formal protocol is in place for fairly addressing employee complaints and disagreements. The larger the hospital, the more important this becomes. Lack of a formal system in this arena could indicate a poorly managed clinic.

15. ***How do you handle unreasonable clients? Do you ever fire clients? How is that decision made?*** While dealing with people is certainly one of the more challenging aspects of being a veterinarian, it isn't too often that you'll encounter an objectively unreasonable, inexcusably rude, intolerably inappropriate, or over-demanding client, but it will

happen. A practice that allows its staff to be mistreated by the public is not a place you want to work.

16. ***What is the typical weekly schedule for the doctors here? On average, how many hours a week do they work? Are there on-call duties after hours and if so, how are they compensated?*** If the schedule is 9 to 5 Monday through Friday with no after hours or weekend duties, and the practice is a pleasant place to work, take the job. Unfortunately, I don't think this schedule exists for veterinarians. A more likely schedule for a GP veterinarian is 7 or 8AM to 6 or 7PM, four days a week plus a half Saturday every other week. And don't forget, medical records, client callbacks and last minute, walk-in emergencies can easily keep you at the hospital beyond closing. If there are no after hours on-call duties, and it's a pleasant place to work, this can be sustainable if you don't have children or pets. If you do, you need a great support system to care for them while you're at work.

Keep in mind that standard full-time employment is 40 hours per week. If you worked 9 to 5 Monday through Friday, with an hour for lunch every day, you'd have time to exercise in the morning, have a leisurely lunch, stop at the grocery store on your way home and make dinner every night. You'd have one weekend day to perform chores and errands like grocery shopping, and house and yard work, and another day off to relax and engage in fun and fulfilling activities.

But if your work week consists of 10 to 12 hour days, four days a week, and another 5 to 6 hours every other Saturday, depending on the culture of your hospital and how stressful your days are at work, you could conceivably find yourself too exhausted to manage non-work related responsibilities and take care of yourself when you do have time off.

If this is the schedule you accept, the salary you're offered should be higher depending on how stressful the environment is. If you work at a place that wears you down every day, your salary should enable you to pay your expenses, including your student loan payments, save, eat out several times a week, have money left over for entertainment and fun – and it should also allow you to hire someone else to clean your house, mow your lawn and walk your dogs – because you won't have the energy to do these things.

Regarding after-hours and on-call duties, if you're in an urban or suburban area where after-hours ER hospitals are accessible, and this hospital still expects you to be on-call, you are nothing but a revenue generator to them. Run, don't walk, to the nearest exit. I once interviewed at a hospital that employed an overnight technician, but not an overnight doctor. There were plenty of 24/7 ERs in the area but this hospital wanted to increase its revenue by offering "monitored" 24/7 care. Doctors were discouraged from referring patients who needed 24/7 care and instead were expected to take calls in the middle of the night for the patients they hospitalized (with no additional compensation). This hospital did not prioritize the best interests of the patients, or of the doctors, and not for a million dollars would I work there.

If you're in a rural community without an emergency hospital, you will likely need to share on-call duties with the other doctors. If this is the case, there should be additional compensation for every after-hours case you see. I'm not asking you to become a mercenary. I know you don't want to be a veterinarian for the money. You want to be a veterinarian so you can help animals. But this doesn't mean you should allow yourself to be exploited and worked to death. You are a human being with errands to run and bills to pay like everyone else, and you need and deserve to have a life outside of work. A good employer will recognize this and their policies will reflect that.

17. ***Are there additional responsibilities for doctors outside of work, such as needing to attend events for hospital promotion? Are the doctors compensated for their time at these events?***
Veterinary hospitals need to engage in marketing

themselves to the community, and some do participate in community events such as parades or fairs. Ideally, your participation as a doctor at these events should be voluntary. If your participation is mandatory, you should be compensated for your time.

18. *If employee meetings are scheduled for a day when I'm off-duty, can I call into the meeting?* This is especially important to ask if the hospital is a long distance from your home. Knowing in advance whether you will be expected to be physically present for employee meetings on your days off is something to take into consideration before accepting the position.

19. *How long do the doctors get for lunch?* As an ER vet without a set schedule, you eat lunch or dinner or a midnight snack when you can. That's the nature of the beast, so this isn't a question I'd ask when applying for an ER position. As a GP though, I wouldn't accept anything less than an hour for lunch. In the real world, where doctors often end up behind schedule because of the unforeseeable and the uncontrollable, anything less than an hour is frequently going to mean you won't get a break at all. Questions 20 - 26 are also only pertinent to an interview for a GP position.

20. ***How long are appointments?*** A good answer is that appointment time varies depending on the reason for the visit. A wellness appointment may be 15 or 20 minutes. A pet who's coming in because he's sick should be given a longer appointment. If every appointment is 15 minutes or less, your days are going to be unpleasant, to say the least. In a hospital running at 100% efficiency, with superb and plentiful support staff, and enough exam rooms for you to juggle at least three appointments simultaneously (this means a minimum of three exam rooms per doctor working on any given day), it may be possible for you to practice good quality care, but few hospitals that I've seen fit this description. The best hospitals I've worked at have 30 minute appointments, with flexibility for scheduling more time if the doctor feels it necessary.

21. ***How often do doctors get double or triple booked?*** I've heard of hospitals that will double and triple book 15 minute appointment slots for their doctors. There is no way any doctor can practice good medicine under these circumstances, no matter how experienced. Sometimes it may be necessary to double book an appointment slot if a client calls in with an emergency – however – a good hospital will ask the doctor's permission before double booking an

appointment slot, giving the doctor the opportunity to say no and direct the client to the nearest emergency hospital.

22. ***If a doctor thinks a certain patient is going to need more time than what they've been scheduled for, can that doctor ask the receptionist to reschedule the appointment for a longer time?*** The answer you want to this question is "yes." Responsibility without authority causes stress. You are going to have a lot of responsibility as a doctor. If a hospital isn't willing to give you the authority to decide when a patient needs more of your time, trust me, you will not be happy there.

23. ***Will I be given more time for my appointments until I get up to speed?*** The answer you want to this question is obviously "yes." Preferably, they will offer some detail as to how much time you'll be given in the beginning and how it will be determined when you're ready to take on a full schedule.

24. ***How are walk-ins and drop-offs handled?*** There are hospitals that double and triple book 15 minute appointment slots, and expect these doctors to also see an unlimited number of drop-offs and walk-ins. Hospitals like this are driven to make as much money as possible for the hospital owner. They aren't interested in providing high quality medical care, nor are they interested in the psychological health of

their employees. When you ask this question, you want to hear that drop-offs are limited to a reasonable number per day, and ideally, you want to hear that doctor discretion governs how many drop-offs and walk-ins will be seen.

25. **What is your hospital's policy on clients who call right before closing wanting to have their pets seen?** A good hospital leaves this up to doctors' discretion. If there are no ER hospitals in your area, obviously the day practices have to provide after-hours care, but if there are emergency animal hospitals available, then the doctor at the day practice should be able to decide, based on the circumstances, whether he or she will wait for a client who wants to come in at the last minute before closing (which usually ends up being *after* closing). If the hospital has a policy that anyone calling at any time must be seen, and the doctor has no say In the matter, this is unlikely to be a hospital where doctors feel respected and happy.

26. **How are the doctors scheduled for surgery?** The best hospital I worked at had doctors rotate surgery duties by the day of the week, and surgeries were performed in the morning before lunch, with the number of surgeries (including dentals) being limited to two (unless a pet with severe periodontal disease was scheduled for a dental, in which case, since these are extremely time consuming, no other procedure

would be scheduled that day). Allowing two hours per elective surgery is very reasonable. Remember, surgery includes the time it takes to perform a pre-operative physical exam, to draw, run and review blood work, to design a pre-anesthetic plan, to induce, shave and prep the patient, to perform the surgery itself, to recover the patient afterwards, to update the client, to write discharge instructions, to prescribe post-operative medications, and to write a surgical record. Some hospitals have doctors rotate surgery days and the doctor performing surgery on a particular day performs surgeries all day, and sees no appointments. This is fine, so long as surgical procedures are limited to a reasonable number.

27. **What are your anesthetic and surgical protocols?** First of all, they should have them. If they don't, ask if they'd be open to collaborating with you to develop them or if you'd be given free rein to use the protocols of your choice. This can be considered another way of asking whether you would be allowed to adhere to your own standards of care.

28. **What kind of pain medications do you carry?** You'll learn more about this subject in your pharmacology class in vet school, but for now I'm just going to say I wouldn't work at any hospital that doesn't carry injectable, full-opioid pain medications like morphine, hydromorphone or oxymorphone. If buprenorphine (a partial opioid and a less effective analgesic) is the

best injectable pain medication they've got, and they're not willing to get full opioids on your request, this says the administration at this hospital considers it too much trouble to go through the process of getting DEA approval to carry good pain medications for their patients.

29. ***Do you ever use relief vets?*** This is a sneaky way of finding out how they handle doctor absences, whether for vacation or illness or whatever. If they have a policy of not using relief vets, guess who fills in when another doctor needs to take time off? Unless they tell you the practice owner covers all absences, most likely, it's going to be you. Also, a practice that refuses to use relief vets is unlikely to be sympathetic or supportive when one of their doctors is sick or has a family emergency. They may offer all sorts of seemingly benevolent explanations for why they don't use relief vets - 'we feel our own doctors are going to provide the best care to our clients and their pets,' or something to that effect. The more likely reason is that they don't want to have to pay for relief vets.

30. ***What's your referral policy?*** If the interviewer tells you they like to handle as much as they can in-house, unless they have board certified specialists on staff, this is a giant, red flag. Even if you're in a rural area, as the doctor, you should have carte blanche to refer

when you feel it's appropriate – even if the nearest specialty hospital is hours away. If you need someone else's approval to refer a case, this hospital is more interested in making money than empowering its doctors to provide quality medical care. This has nothing to do with whether a client is willing or able to pursue a specialty consult. This is purely about whether you are able to recommend referal when you believe it's warranted.

31. ***How do you deal with client financial constraints? Do you ever discount services? Do you offer Care Credit or some kind of payment plan?*** What you're really asking here is how much flexibility you have as a doctor when confronting the financial limits of a client. I don't advocate providing discounted or free services because this leads to inappropriate client demands and expectations. You'll meet some clients who can afford medical care for their pets but would rather not pay for it if they can help it, and they will try to bully and guilt you into providing discounts. They will accuse you of being greedy and of not caring about animals. Discounted and free services are not for them.

Veterinary hospitals have to be profitable. If they aren't, you won't have a job, and medical care won't be available to any pet. Veterinary hospitals have expenses - they buy costly medical equipment and drugs and supplies, they have electricity bills and software licensing fees and employees to pay -

employees who have families to support. Clients who try to emotionally blackmail or manipulate veterinarians, are in my experience, not the type of clients who truly cannot afford medical care for their pets. I feel profoundly sorry for animals who belong to people like this, but I cannot give in to this kind of manipulation. If I discounted or gave away my services to everyone who tried this tactic on me, my hospital would go bankrupt and I would be living under a bridge and using fragments of rubber tires collected off the highway as fuel to cook Ramen noodles.

However, I have met some genuinely good people who genuinely loved their pets and were genuinely heartbroken they could not afford medical care for their beloved companions. These people were courteous and polite. They did not blame me for the unfortunate circumstance they found themselves in. In my experience, truly poor people do not demand services for free, and they are kind and thankful for any small thing you do to help them. For these people, I will bend over backwards to try to find some sort of solution.

One way of distinguishing between someone who has money but doesn't want to spend it - from someone who would spend money to help their own pet if only they had it - is whether they are willing to apply for Care Credit. Care Credit is like a credit card for health expenses that people can apply for on the spot, and an answer is often received within thirty minutes or less as to whether a line of credit has been approved. People who have money but don't want to spend it will refuse to apply for Care Credit - because they know they're likely to be approved - and then they can't claim to have no money. People who genuinely don't have the funds to pay for medical care for their pets will be happy to apply for Care Credit, and will keep their fingers crossed that they are approved.

At the ER where I worked, we used this as a litmus test. If clients claiming to have no money agreed to apply for Care Credit, even if they were declined, that gave us an idea of how genuine they were. If they tried calling friends and relatives to borrow money, if they were courteous and polite, we would do something to help them - it wouldn't be Gold Standard Veterinary Medicine - it couldn't be - but it would be something.

This is the flexibility you want as a doctor. You want to have the discretion to help the genuinely good people who genuinely love their pets - in some way. You're not going to bankrupt the hospital by just giving an injection of an antibiotic and sending home a couple of pain killers, or giving some subcutaneous fluids, or by performing a free euthanasia on a suffering animal once in a while. Does the hospital where you're interviewing have Care Credit? Will they allow you to use your own discretion? Or do they have a clause in their contract stating that if you discount services or do anything for free you are committing theft and will be charged and fired? I'm not exaggerating. I have seen contracts like this.

32. **_Do you ever allow relinquishment?_** This, like the last question, is about how much flexibility you would be given as a doctor at this hospital. Some hospitals allow doctors to offer owners who can't afford needed medical care for their pets to relinquish that pet to the hospital (just like I offered relinquishment to Rhoda's owner). The hospital then provides the needed medical care and finds a new home for the animal. For example, a young, otherwise healthy dog may present with bloat. Without surgery he will die, but the owner can't afford it. If this dog were thirteen years old, surgery might not make practical sense, but in this case the surgery would likely mean many more good years of life for this dog.

An owner who is truly interested in the best interests of his dog will give up ownership in order to grant those extra years of life to an animal he loves. If you worked at this hospital, would you have the right to offer that option if you felt moved to do so? If the interviewer's answer is "no," this isn't necessarily a deal-breaker. Some hospitals truly don't have the resources to take on this responsibility. On the other hand, what if you, the doctor, wanted to take on this responsibility yourself? What if you took on ownership and the job of finding a new home for this animal? What if you performed or paid for the treatment yourself? You'll want the answers to these questions before deciding whether or not you want to work there.

33. ***What's your stance on convenience euthanasia or is this up to the individual doctor?*** Convenience euthanasia means the owner wants to euthanize his pet for a reason that does not warrant euthanasia. I think the purpose of this question is clear enough. What you make of the interviewer's answer is a matter of personal ethics.

What Employers
Want From You

Employment is a two-way street. While you want to avoid working in a bad hospital, you also want to make yourself desirable to, and worthy of, a good hospital. According to a 2009 article in the Journal of Veterinary Medical Education, "Most employers regarded employing and training new graduates to be financially and personally costly, commenting that It takes six to 12 months (and sometimes up to 24 months) for a graduate to earn their salary in terms of professional fees."[5] When a good hospital hires a new graduate, they are providing the additional training you need after veterinary school, paying you a much better salary than what you'd get as an intern, and asking less of you than an internship would.

Why? Because they see potential in you and they're hoping you'll stay, at least long enough to justify their investment. If you leave within two or three years, it's a "significant drain on the human and financial resources" of the practice.[5] While I want to see the field of veterinary medicine brimming over with happy and successful veterinarians, I also want to see a proliferation of good animal hospitals, and that requires the good hospitals to be profitable. Here are a few things you can do to make yourself a good investment to a good hospital.

Stay. It seems like the whole world is on fast forward these days. Change has always been a constant, but the rate of change seems to have accelerated drastically in the last two decades. I find it difficult to make commitments for the future because today could bring any number of surprises that may compel me to change those plans. Promising to stay in one place for five years seems inconceivable, but ideally you will stay at your first practice for at least that long. I won't ask you to stay anywhere you feel unhappy, disrespected, exploited, or unappreciated. If however you are lucky enough to land your first job in one of those good hospitals where they do provide mentorship, where they practice good medicine, where they treat you like a human being who needs to have a life outside of work... If at all possible, do your best to ensure their success and to repay their investment in you, and stay at least five years.

Survey says... A survey of small animal practice owners published in 2004 yielded a list of procedures considered most important for new graduates to be able to perform competently.[7] Here I list the top 15 in order of frequency rank. These are skills expected of new GP veterinarians, although ER vets should be proficient at numbers 1, 2, 10, and 15. If you can walk in the door on day one of being a GP veterinarian and feel comfortable doing these things, you'll be in good shape. As discussed earlier though, much of the knowledge and many of the skills needed by GP veterinarians won't be emphasized in veterinary school. You'll need to be proactive during your clinical rotations to achieve competence of these skills.

1. Routine venipuncture
2. Induction of anesthesia, intubation and maintenance of anesthesia
3. Anal sac expression
4. Vaccination protocols and techniques
5. Castration
6. Ovariohysterectomy
7. Ear cleaning
8. Dental prophylaxis
9. Heartworm testing
10. Wound management
11. Peripheral venous catheter placement
12. Tooth extraction
13. Skin scraping for mites
14. Onychectomy
15. Cystocentesis

Don't expect to work as hard as the experienced doctors. Expect to work harder. I mentioned earlier that you should expect to stay late until your learn to effectively manage your time as a practitioner, but even after you master the art of getting out on time, a great portion of the time after hours should be devoted to identifying and filling your knowledge gaps. Keep your veterinary textbooks. Buy more. Read them. Scour the medical literature. No one is going to assign you extra reading or ask that you make presentations to demonstrate your increasing medical knowledge, and you won't have the impetus of impending exams to drive you. The benefit of not doing a residency is better pay and better hours. The cost is that you must be a proactive and wholly self-directed learner.

Be a great mentee. Don't expect your mentors to do the heavy lifting. They're making sacrifices for your benefit just by agreeing to mentor you. You need to do your part. Be proactive. Identify your weaknesses. Decide for yourself what your learning objectives should be and how you think you'll best achieve them. Design your own mentorship plan. After you've done this work, then ask for feedback on your plan. Make sure you know what they expect of you and that they feel comfortable with your expectations of them. Recognize this is an iterative process. As you grow, you'll identify new areas for improvement and the process will begin again. Schedule regular meetings based on your mentors' availability. These meeting are to keep you accountable, to discuss your progress and to agree on the next objectives.

Another way to be a great mentee is to know how to frame your clinical questions. Inexperienced doctors have a tendency to give too much information when they're asking a clinical question of a more experienced colleague. I was guilty of this myself. I thought the more information I gave, the better. I didn't want to leave anything important out. But retrospectively I realize I was doing this because I hadn't taken the time beforehand to think critically about what I was asking. I just brain-dumped all over them. Your mentors are busy. They don't have time for a fifteen minute hallway chat. So before you approach them with a question, first figure out what the real question is, and then provide only the minimum information they need to help you answer that question.

In vet school you'll be taught to present cases like this: "This is a ten year old, male, neutered Cocker Spaniel with a history of food allergies but doing well on a duck and potato diet. He is presenting today for lethargy, inappetance and intermittent vomiting. Physical exam findings reveal normal TPR, a body condition score of 8 out of 10, bilateral lenticular sclerosis, ceruminous debris AU (in both ears), mild discomfort on upper right abdominal palpation, and jaundice. Blood work shows a PCV of 45%, normal white blood cell count, an ALT of 98 u/L, ALK Phos of 176 u/L, AST of 34 u/L (these are liver enzymes), and bilirubin of 2.5. Recommend abdominal ultrasound focusing on the liver and gall bladder."

Ain't nobody got time for that in the real world! First of all, the problem here is likely the gall bladder or liver. The dog's history of food allergies, what he eats and the physical exam findings about being overweight, lens thickening (normal in an older dog) and a little gunk in his ears with no signs of inflammation or discomfort are not pertinent. Let's say what you want to ask in this case is for the senior clinician to help you perform an ultrasound to look at the dog's liver and gallbladder.

Just say, "I've got an old, jaundiced Cocker Spaniel with acute vomiting, moderately elevated liver enzymes and a bilirubin of 2.5. His PCV is normal. Can you help me perform an ultrasound?" (Including information about the normal PCV, which is a measure of red blood cell count, is important because immune mediated hemolytic anemia or IMHA causes red blood cell destruction and that can also cause the yellowing of the skin called jaundice – so a normal red blood cell count indicates IMHA isn't the problem. Don't worry. You'll know stuff like this when you start practicing.)

A quick tip in all cases is to begin with the problem (for example, a jaundiced, vomiting dog), then give the minimum information you think is relevant, then ask your question. This will feel a little uncomfortable when you're new because you won't feel wholly confident about which medical details are essential and which aren't. Resist the urge to brain-dump on your mentor, take a moment to think critically and err on the side of breviloquence. If the senior clinician thinks more information is needed in order to answer your question, she'll ask.

In additional to your mentor, other people you can call on for help with your cases include doctors at nearby emergency or specialty hospitals, your vet school professors and consultants at outside laboratories like Idexx, Antech and Abaxis. Often specialists employed at these labs will answer your questions for free, especially if your hospital uses their services regularly. These outside labs also offer more in-depth medical consults for a fee for the more complex medical cases.

Avoid mentee pitfalls. New doctors are filled with angst and self-doubt yet simultaneously feel as if they must appear flawless. According to a 2017 article in the *Journal of the American Medical Association*, these feelings can lead to counterproductive patterns of behavior that can potentially harm their relationship with mentors, as well as their future careers. The article lists six predictable negative patterns of behavior mentees should actively avoid:[20]

> **Over committing:** As a new doctor, you'll be eager to prove yourself. You'll want to say yes to every challenge, "regardless of relevance or benefit" to your career. Saying yes to everything gives others the perception that you have the capacity to take on more, and more will be asked of you. Eventually this will lead to "high-output

failure typified by diminishing quantity and quality" of your work. Only you know what your true capacity is, and it's your responsibility to say no when a new request exceeds that capacity. It's better to under-promise and over-deliver than to overpromise and under-deliver.

Being a doormat: The doormat not only says yes to every challenge, he also says yes to being used as a tool for making someone else's job easier - to his own detriment. It may beneficial for a mentee to run all the lab work and print and fill every prescription for a week or two. This can be justified as providing the mentee with the logistical training that will ultimately make him more effective in the practice. But the doormat will continue to perform someone else's scutwork indefinitely. To avoid being a doormat, you've got to have the courage to diplomatically say no to work that is inappropriate for you. This doesn't mean you shouldn't clean a cage every now and then when the situation calls for it. It means recognizing when you're being continuously taken advantage of and standing up for yourself.

Ghosting: Ghosting is avoidance. It's trying to stay out of sight of a mentor, especially when the mentee is concerned her performance may not be up to par. She tries to remain out of sight in hopes her poor performance will be forgotten or will go unnoticed. This behavior dooms the mentee-mentor relationship to mutual distrust. If you make an error or feel you may not be living up to expectations, you've got to do the opposite of what your instincts may tell you to do. Instead of hiding, come out. The most impressive thing a new doctor can do is to be honest about her own perceived shortcomings, to own up to a mistake or to ask for advice on how she can improve her performance.

Being a vampire: One of the most daunting aspects of being a new doctor is making decisions. Should you prescribe this antibiotic or a different one? Should you prescribe an antibiotic at all? Should you ignore a minor abnormality on blood work or should you follow it up with more tests? In the beginning, you're going to want your mentor's validation of every little decision you make. Resist this urge. Don't hound your mentor when you're both in the hospital. Don't barrage your mentor with "countless emails, text messages, phone calls, and meeting requests." Remember your mentor is a busy doctor with his own responsibilities and his own cases to work up. Accept the burden of decision making that belongs to every doctor. Learn to discriminate between decisions unlikely to lead to harm and decisions that may have serious consequences. The latter require guidance and warrant interrupting your mentor. The former don't. In cases of low-risk decisions, use books, medical websites and your own knowledge. You can save questions related to these cases for a later time when you're scheduled to meet with your mentor.

Being a lone wolf: I was a lone wolf. The lone wolf appears confident and seems to need no help or guidance. She proceeds boldly on her own. This affect however masks an underlying fear of asking for help lest she seem "weak or foolish." This behavior becomes her undoing when a "preventable but highly embarrassing error occurs due to lack of guidance." The lone wolf is the opposite of the vampire, but the solution is the same. Always take the time to ask yourself: "Does this decision have the potential for serious consequences?" If the answer is yes, ask for guidance before proceeding.

Backstabbing: When your own inner dialogue, that nasty backseat driver, is already beating you up all day, every day, it's hard to accept criticism from outside sources as well. When you're doing the best you can under less than ideal conditions, such as feeling hurried or being under staffed, and something goes wrong, it's tempting to want to place the blame elsewhere. Perhaps a technician was at fault, or it's your mentor's fault for not being there when you needed her, or it's because some other doctor told you to do it that way... While all those things may be true, never use excuses or blame others to shield yourself from the responsibility that is ultimately yours alone. Fair or not, you are the doctor and you are responsible. Accept the blame and learn from the error, no matter whose error it was.

Logistical Advice

Following are a few pieces of miscellaneous logistical advice that will be helpful to know before you begin practicing:

Continuing education

Every veterinary doctor is required to complete a specific number of continuing education hours. This number varies by state. In Illinois, the CE requirement for veterinarians is 40 hours every two years. In Arizona, the requirement is 20 hours every two years. Employers usually (and should) provide a yearly CE allowance for their veterinarians. My first employer offered $2,000 per year for my CE allowance. I could use this money for CE conferences held anywhere in the country, or the world. I could use it for subscriptions to medical journals, or for textbooks, or anything that safely fell into the category of furthering my own medical education.

Depending on the state where you begin working, most new veterinary graduates are exempt from having to attain CE credits their first year out of school. My medical director advised me not to wait however and so I used my first year's CE allowance to attend the VECCS (Veterinary Emergency & Critical Care Society) CE conference in San Antonio. Including the conference costs, airfare, hotel, and meals, I spent over $3,000 on that trip. Travelling out of town for CE conferences is exciting and fun but, depending on the nature of the CE, not necessarily justifiable in an economic sense.

Multi-day CE conferences are intellectually draining as well. You'll want to go to every lecture you can fit into your schedule, but you'll soon find that your brain can only effectively absorb so much information in a day. I didn't feel I could get my money's worth out of that conference because I was intellectually exhausted after the first day. Because of this, as well as the added cost of travel, I wouldn't advise using your CE allowance for out of town conferences. If you become an AVMA member after you graduate, as of this writing, your first AVMA CE Conference is free. Ideally, you'll attend this conference for the first time when it's scheduled within driving distance of where you live.

There are plenty of online resources for veterinary CE that you can complete at your leisure, at home, in your pajamas. Some are even free. Just make sure the courses you take for CE credit are "RACE Approved." RACE is a stamp of approval indicating the courses meet minimum standards for veterinary continuing education. Go to www.realize.vet/book3-resources for a list. Additionally, state and city veterinary medical associations, as well as local specialty hospitals, frequently offer CE courses throughout the year - for little to no cost.

Aside from your desire to just have fun and enjoy the camaraderie and excitement of being at a big veterinary CE conference despite the costs, the only other exception I would make in terms of traveling out of town for veterinary CE would be if you wanted to attend the hands-on laboratory continuing education courses offered at the Oquendo Center in Las Vegas, Nevada.

Class sizes are small so you'll get direct guidance, and they offer practical education on important topics such as "Top Ten Surgical Procedures," "Ophthalmic Surgery for the General Practitioner," "Comprehensive Small Animal Dentistry," as well as courses on ultrasound and endoscopy. This kind of hands-on supervised training will benefit you more than a hundred lectures. In fact, if you can swing it financially, I would suggest taking one of their surgery courses before you even begin practicing.

State Laws

While every veterinarian has to pass the NAVLE (North American Veterinary Licensing Examination) before they can become licensed to practice in the United States, some states will also require you to pass an examination before granting you a state license. I didn't have to sit for a state exam to get my Illinois license, but I did have to pass an exam to get licensed in Arizona. Additionally, all states have their own statutes and administrative rules governing the practice of veterinary medicine. The best place to get information on state licensing procedures and state regulations is from the state veterinary medical board. Search for the state's "Veterinary Practice Act." Regardless of whether the state you plan to practice in has an exam, it's important for you to familiarize yourself with that state's procedures and statutes. This is where you'll find out how many CE hours are required, how the board is structured, what the protocols are for board complaints, what procedures certified technicians can and cannot legally perform in that state, and other important information governing the practice of veterinary medicine in your state.

State License(s)

If you start practicing in Florida because that's where you got the best job offer, but your family lives in Delaware and you know someday you want to go back there, get licensed in both Florida and Delaware as soon as you graduate. Maintain your CE hours according to both states, and pay your licensing fees for both states every year (licensing fees for vets are usually a couple hundred dollars every couple of years). Most states, if not all, will allow you to obtain a veterinary medical license (either with or without a state exam) without re-taking the NAVLE if you passed the NAVLE within the past 5 years. After that time period, if you want to get licensed in another state, you have to re-take the NAVLE. Taking the NAVLE is stressful enough as a veterinary student because it asks questions about so many different species. At least as a veterinary student, all that information is fresh in your mind. Five years out of school, however, after you've practiced nothing but small animal medicine, having to re-take the NAVLE will mean having to relearn all that stuff about horses and pigs and cows and chickens that you've long forgotten.

To DEA or Not to DEA

You will be allowed to prescribe controlled substances to your patients using your hospital's DEA number *if* what you're prescribing is dispensed from your hospital. However, if you want to prescribe a controlled substance that your hospital doesn't carry, you need your own DEA license to write that prescription. There's also always a possibility of an inventory oversight that results in your hospital running out of a controlled substance. For example, if you need to refill an epileptic patient's phenobarbital but your hospital has run out of this drug, you can write a prescription that can be filled at an outside pharmacy – *if* you have your own DEA license.

Therefore, despite the cost (as of this writing, the cost for a DEA license is $750 every two years), I recommend getting your own DEA license. Some employers will cover this cost for their veterinarians. When I was close to graduating, I started thinking about things like state and

DEA licenses. I asked my pharmacology professor what I needed to do in order to get my DEA license. He had no idea! After I got my state license, I emailed the State Veterinary Medical Board in Illinois to ask them how to get a DEA license. They never answered. I'm sure they thought that was the dumbest question ever. But if it was such a dumb question, how come a pharmacology professor at a vet school didn't know? Let me save you the stress and aggravation. It actually is straightforward - once you figure it out! First get your state veterinary medical license, then fill out the online application. Google *new DEA license* or get the direct link via my website at www.realize.vet/book3-resources

Zoonoses

When I see a veterinary patient with a nasty skin infection, a productive cough or bloody diarrhea, I don't cringe with disgust. I would if my patients were humans. Sick people are indisputably more yucky than sick animals, to me at least. I suspect the evolutionary explanation for this is feeling revolted by signs of illness in another human being grants me a survival advantage. By avoiding that human, I'm less likely to catch something contagious.

However, instincts and personal preferences aside, when it comes to contagious diseases, I have almost as much to fear from my animal patients as Alex has to fear from his human patients. 61% of human pathogens and

75% of emerging diseases that affect humans are zoonotic, meaning they are transmissible between humans and other animals. Currently, there are greater than 50 important zoonotic diseases in the United States.[21] The National Association of State Public Health Veterinarians (NASPHV) published a *Compendium of Veterinary Standard Precautions for Zoonotic Disease Prevention in Veterinary Personnel in 2015*. You can obtain this document with an internet search or via direct link from www.realize.vet/book3-resources

It will be your duty, as a veterinarian, to ensure proper precautions are being taken to protect yourself, your family, your staff, your patients, and your clients – even if you're not a practice owner. I can't stress enough the importance of reading this document before you begin practicing, but here I will at least relay the NASPHV recommendations for inoculations.

> ***Rabies.*** Veterinarians, veterinary students and veterinary support staff are in a high-risk category for exposure to the deadly rabies virus. Most, if not all, veterinary schools require vet students to get pre-exposure rabies vaccinations. (A 2013 survey of US veterinary schools revealed that only 1 of the 21 responding schools did *not* require pre-exposure immunization for rabies of its students.)[16] The advantage of pre-exposure rabies immunization is - if you're exposed to the virus - you won't need to get the painful series of post-exposure rabies immunoglobulin injections.

Rabies immunoglobulins are antibodies that come from either horses or humans who have high numbers of antibodies in their blood. These immunoglobulin injections are painful because large quantities, usually about 10ml, must be injected into a muscle. These immunoglobulin injections also cost thousands of dollars. If you're exposed to a potentially rabid animal, and you received pre-exposure inoculation, you can forego this costly nightmare. You'll only need another series of the regular rabies vaccine, but these are 1ml injections.

Rabies vaccination of veterinary personnel is not legally required,[12] although for obvious reasons, it is recommended by the NASPHV, the U.S. Centers for Disease Control and the World Health Organization. If your veterinary school does not require rabies vaccination, read the CDC's Rabies VIS (Vaccination Information Statement) that you can search for online or obtain via direct link from
www.realize.vet/book3-resources
- then talk to your doctor or contact your local or state health department for information on getting pre-exposure rabies immunization. After you have been vaccinated, get your serum rabies antibody titers checked every two years. If the laboratory determines the titers are too low to be protective, you will need a booster.[3]

Tetanus. The CD recommends tetanus vaccination every ten years for everyone. It may be even more important for veterinary personnel however since animal bites are "tetanus-prone wounds."[21] Tetanus is a serious, painful and potentially fatal disease caused by toxins that are produced by the bacterial species Clostridium tetani. These toxins can cause muscle spasms severe enough to fracture your bones and break your back. If you sustain a wound that could lead to tetanus and you are not up to date on your tetanus vaccine, you will need an injection of tetanus immune globulin. Like the rabies immunoglobulin injections, the tetanus immune globulin injection is painful because large quantities (12-24ml) of the solution must be injected directly into a muscle.

Influenza. The CDC recommends yearly vaccination against the flu for everyone older than six months. If you're young and healthy, you may feel this is an unnecessary precaution for you. (Although it may interest you to know that some influenza viruses, such as the strain implicated in the influenza pandemic of 1918, can cause even more serious signs of illness in people with healthy immune systems.) Regardless, no matter the virus strain, what typically characterizes the flu is that it debilitates you. It's not "the sniffles," or a persistent and inconvenient cough, or even a mild fever with a few minor aches. If it's the genuine article, the flu will knock you off your feet and keep you horizontal for several days, and I don't know anyone (except for mothers of small children) less able to take sick days than a veterinarian. However, perhaps the most important reason to get an annual flu vaccine is to protect the other people you come into contact with, especially clients who are elderly or may be immune-compromised.

You Are Amazing

I know I've packed this book full of all kinds of potentially overwhelming information. Kudos to you for getting this far. There's one last little story I want to tell you though, and I hope you'll bear with me, because this is really important for you to know.

After over two years of working as an overnight ER veterinarian, I still felt inadequate. At that time Alex was working his way through his Internal Medicine residency. As a resident, he was required to work overnights several weeks a year, and during those short periods, our schedules were compatible. One morning during one of those periods, after we had both returned from our overnight shifts, I told him about the horrific night I'd had. I told him how I felt I couldn't do anything right, about how vexed and befuddled I was about a particular case, how demoralized I felt.

"Oh you DVMs," he said to me, shaking his head. "Why do a 3-year residency in Internal Medicine, a 5-year residency in Emergency Medicine, a 5-year residency in Radiology, and a 6-year residency in Surgery, when you can just graduate from medical school and do all of those things simultaneously from day 1? You guys should have as your emblem a picture of a gigantic pair of testicles. You are amazing."

Veterinarians are amazing. Not only are we expected to be able to practice medicine on every kind of animal, we're expected to be proficient in every medical specialty – specialties that require multiple years of residency training for human medical doctors. Any sensible person would agree these expectations are unrealistic, yet most veterinarians continue to strive for this impossible medical omni-competence, and then judge themselves ruthlessly for failing to achieve what is objectively unachievable.

In the book *Complications* by the MD surgeon Atul Gawande, he writes about doctors, "It isn't reasonable to ask that we achieve perfection. What is reasonable is to ask that we never cease to aim for it." Dr. Gawande is a surgeon at Brigham and Women's Hospital, which is adjacent to, and affiliated with, Harvard Medical School. If an MD with years of residency training and experience in his specialty, practicing only his specialty, working in a well-staffed, well-funded, top notch U.S. hospital cannot achieve perfection, what are the chances of achieving perfection for a veterinarian who has to assume the role of multiple specialists despite inadequate knowledge and expertise, and who is working with far fewer resources and under far less ideal conditions?

When you start your career as a veterinarian and begin beating yourself up for not being the perfect doctor you think you ought to be, let this provide a sense of perspective. No matter how badly you think you're doing, remember that being a veterinarian is really, *really* hard. You are doing the best you can to measure up to impossibly high standards under very challenging circumstances. You will work harder than ever before in your life, harder than any of your friends who aren't veterinarians. You will worry more than you've ever worried before. You will suffer when your patients suffer, a part of you will die when your patients die, and you will carry the burden of remorse for every perceived failure. Yet, for the sake of your patients, you will persist and never cease to aim for perfection. You deserve to have a star in the heavens named after you. You are amazing. And you absolutely deserve to have the life you envision for yourself.

For a list of recommended reading related to the topics in this book, go to www.realize.vet/book3-resources

If you found this book helpful, I'd really appreciate if you would leave a positive review where you purchased it online.

Thank you for giving me the privilege of sharing what I know to enhance your experiences as you make the same journey to become a veterinarian that I made years ago. If you have comments or suggestions for improving any of the books in this series, or if you have additional questions you would like to see addressed on my blog or on my podcast, please fill out the survey at www.realize.vet/survey

I wish you a bright and fantastic future as a well prepared and fully empowered Doctor of Veterinary Medicine.

Kindest regards,
Dr. K
Flagstaff, Arizona

Index

1. Albers, John, W. "The Future of Specialty Practice." Journal of Veterinary Medical Education. 2008. (35)1.
2. Burns, Katie. " Recession Leads to Decrease in Revenues at Many Specialty Practices Across the Country." JAVMA News.
3. Fowler, Heather, N., VMD, MPH, et al. " Survey of Occupational Hazards in Minnesota Veterinary Practices in 2012." *Journal of the American Veterinary Medical Association.* January 15, 2016. Volume 248, Number 2.
4. Geller, Jon, DVM, DAVBP. "A Call for Internship Quality Control.*" Journal of the American Veterinary Medical Association.* April 15, 2012. Volume 240, Number 8.
5. Gilling, Marg, L. and Parkinson, Timothy, J. " The Transition from Veterinary Student to

Practitioner: A "Make or Break" Period." *Journal of Veterinary Medical Education*. 2009 (36)2.

6. Gordon, Meg, E., Ms, DVM, et al. "Comparison for Long-Term Implications for Five Veterinary Career Tracks." *Journal of the American Veterinary Medication Association.* August 15, 2010. Volume 237, Number 4.

7. Greenfield, Kathy, L., DVM, MS, DACVS, et al. " Frequency of Use of Various Procedures, Skills, and Areas of Knowledge Among Veterinarians in Private Small Animal Exclusive or Predominant Practice and Proficiency Expected of New Veterinary School Graduates." *Journal of the American Veterinary Medical Association* . June 1, 2014. Volume 224, Number 11.

8. Guiducci, Edward, J., JD. " Veterinary Practice Ownership Agreements: Why Are They Important?" *Wild West Veterinary Conference*. Arvada, CO. 2014.

9. Hickey, Maud. "Can Improvisation Be Taught?: A Call for Free Improvisation in Our Schools." *International Journal of Music Education*. 2009. Volume 27(4) 285–299 [(200911)27:4]

10. http://gomerblog.com/2015/06/bright-eyed-med-students/

11. https://en.wikipedia.org/wiki/Four_stages_of_co mpetence

12. https://www.avma.org/KB/Resources/Reference/ Pages/Rabies-pre-exposure-vaccination-titers-veterinarians.aspx

13. Johnson, Cia, L., DVM, MS, et al. "Elements of and Factors Important in Veterinary Hospice." *Journal of the America Veterinary Medical Association.* January 15, 2011. Volume 238, Number 2.

14. Kipperman, Barry, S., DVM, et al. "Factors that Influence Small Animal Veterinarians' Opinions and Actions Regarding Cost of Care and Effects of Economic Limitations on Patient Care and Outcome and Professional Career Satisfaction and Burnout." *Journal of the American Veterinary Medical Association.* April 1, 2017. Volume 250, Number 7.

15. Klein, Sarah. "*Ways Working the Night Shift Hurts Your Health." *Healthy Living*. August 14, 2014

16. Lindenmayer, Joann, M., et al. " Reported Rabies Pre-exposure Immunization of Students at US Colleges of Veterinary Medicine." *Journal of Veterinary Medical Education*. 2013. (40)3.

17. Rishniw, Mark. " Practice Ownership Aspirations Survey—2016." *Veterinary Information Network*. May 9, 2016.

18. Schmidt, H.G, Ph.D, et al. "A Cognitive Perspective on Medical Expertise: Theory and Implications." *Academic Medicine*. October 1990. Volume 55, Number 10.

19. Stone, Elizabeth, A., et al. "A New Model for Companion-Animal Primary Health Care Education. " *Journal of Veterinary Medical Education*. 2012. (39)3.

20. Vaughn, Valerie, MD, MSc, et al. "Mentee Missteps: Tales for the Academic Trenches." Journal of the American Medical Association. February 7, 2017. Volume 317, Number 5.

21. Williams, Carl, J., DVM, DACVPM, Bell, Michael, R., MD, et al. "Compendium of Veterinary Standard Precautions for Zoonotic Disease Prevention in Veterinary Personnel." *Journal of the American Veterinary Medical Association.* December 1, 2015. Volume 247, Number 11.

www.ingramcontent.com/pod-product-compliance
Lightning Source LLC
Chambersburg PA
CBHW060037040426
42331CB00032B/990